Supervisory Skills
for Nurses

4th Edition

By
Gloria York, RN, MAEd

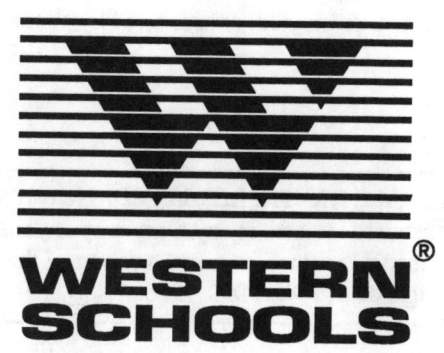

**WESTERN®
SCHOOLS**

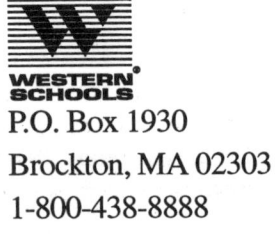

P.O. Box 1930

Brockton, MA 02303

1-800-438-8888

ABOUT THE INSTRUCTIONAL DEVELOPER/EDITOR

Gloria York, R.N., M.A.Ed., is a continuing education development specialist and consultant. Ms. York has been a nurse for over 20 years and has worked as a nurse educator for the last 14 years. She has co-authored guidelines for nursing continuing education, which are now being implemented by several providers around the country. Ms. York has developed numerous instructional products and has published in *The American Journal of Continuing Education in Nursing.* She authored the chapter "Continuing Education for Relicensure" in *Issues and Trends in Nursing,* a Mosby Year Book.

ABOUT THE SUBJECT MATTER EXPERT

Kathy Falkenhagen, RN, BSN, MS, is currently in private practice as President of Nursing Vistas Inc., providing nursing education and consultation on organizational, interpersonal and managerial topics. As a former Director of Surgical Services, Ms. Falkenhagen spent 24 years in the Surgical Services arena at the University of Texas MD Anderson Cancer Center in Houston, Texas. Kathy speaks at conferences, nationally and internationally on numerous leadership and management issues, and belongs to several professional nursing organizations.

Copy Editor: Andrea Posey, RN

Indexer: Sylvia Coates

Typesetter: Kathy Johnson

Western Schools' courses are designed to provide nursing professionals with the educational information they need to enhance their career development. The information provided within these course materials is the result of research and consultation with prominent nursing and medical authorities and is, to the best of our knowledge, current and accurate. However, the courses and course materials are provided with the understanding that Western Schools is not engaged in offering legal, nursing, medical, or other professional advice.

Western Schools' courses and course materials are not meant to act as a substitute for seeking out professional advice or conducting individual research. When the information provided in the courses and course materials is applied to individual circumstances, all recommendations must be considered in light of the uniqueness pertaining to each situation.

Western Schools' course materials are intended solely for *your* use and *not* for the benefit of providing advice or recommendations to third parties. Western Schools devoids itself of any responsibility for adverse consequences resulting from the failure to seek nursing, medical, or other professional advice. Western Schools further devoids itself of any responsibility for updating or revising any programs or publications presented, published, distributed, or sponsored by Western Schools unless otherwise agreed to as part of an individual purchase contract.

ISBN: 1-57801-036-5

IMPORTANT: Read these instructions *BEFORE* proceeding!

Enclosed with your course book you will find the FasTrax® answer sheet. Use this form to answer all the final exam questions that appear in this course book. If you are completing more than one course, be sure to write your answers on the appropriate answer sheet. Full instructions and complete grading details are printed on the FasTrax instruction sheet, also enclosed with your order. Please review them before starting. *If you are mailing your answer sheet(s) to Western Schools, we recommend you make a copy as a backup.*

ABOUT THIS COURSE

A "Pretest" is provided with each course to test your current knowledge base regarding the subject matter contained within this course. Your "Final Exam" is a multiple choice examination. **You will find the exam questions at the end of each chapter.** Some smaller hour courses include the exam at the end of the book.

In the event the course has less than 100 questions, mark your answers to the questions in the course book and leave the remaining answer boxes on the FasTrax answer sheet blank. **Use a black pen to fill in your answer sheet.**

A PASSING SCORE

You must score 70% or better in order to pass this course and receive your Certificate of Completion. Should you fail to achieve the required score, we will send you an additional FasTrax answer sheet so that you may make a second attempt to pass the course. Western Schools will allow you three chances to pass the same course...*at no extra charge!* After three failed attempts to pass the same course, your file will be closed.

RECORDING YOUR HOURS

Please monitor the time it takes to complete this course using the handy log sheet on the other side of this page. See below for transferring study hours to the course evaluation.

COURSE EVALUATIONS

In this course book you will find a short evaluation about the course you are soon to complete. This information is vital to providing the school with feedback on this course. The course evaluation answer section is in the lower right hand corner of the FasTrax answer sheet marked "Evaluation" with answers marked 1–25. Your answers are important to us, please take five minutes to complete the evaluation.

On the back of the FasTrax instruction sheet there is additional space to make any comments about the course, the school, and suggested new curriculum. Please mail the FasTrax instruction sheet, with your comments, back to Western Schools in the envelope provided with your course order.

TRANSFERRING STUDY TIME

Upon completion of the course, transfer the total study time from your log sheet to question #25 in the Course Evaluation. The answers will be in ranges, please choose the proper hour range that best represents your study time. You MUST log your study time under question #25 on the course evaluation.

EXTENSIONS

You have 2 years from the date of enrollment to complete this course. A six (6) month extension may be purchased. If after 30 months from the original enrollment date you do not complete the course, *your file will be closed and no certificate can be issued.*

CHANGE OF ADDRESS?

In the event you have moved during the completion of this course please call our student services department at 1-800-618-1670 and we will update your file.

A GUARANTEE YOU'LL GIVE HIGH HONORS TO

If any continuing education course fails to meet your expectations or if you are not satisfied in any manner, for any reason, you may return it for an exchange or a refund (less shipping and handling) within 30 days. Software, video and audio courses must be returned unopened.

Thank you for enrolling at Western Schools!

WESTERN SCHOOLS
P.O. Box 1930
Brockton, MA 02303
(800) 438-8888
www.westernschools.com

Supervisory Skills for Nurses

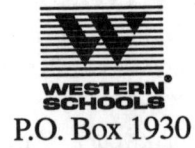

WESTERN SCHOOLS

P.O. Box 1930
Brockton, MA 02303

Please use this log to total the number of hours you spend reading the text and taking the final examination (use 50-min hours).

Date	Hours Spent
_____	_____
_____	_____
_____	_____
_____	_____
_____	_____
_____	_____
_____	_____
_____	_____
_____	_____
_____	_____
_____	_____
_____	_____
_____	_____

TOTAL [   ]

Please log your study hours with submission of your final exam. To log your study time, fill in the appropriate circle under question 25 of the FasTrax® answer sheet under the "Evaluation" section.

Please choose the answer that represents the total study hours it took you to complete this 30 hour course.

A. less than 25 hours

B. 25–28 hours

C. 29–32 hours

D. greater than 32 hours

Supervisory Skills for Nurses

WESTERN SCHOOLS' NURSING
CONTINUING EDUCATION EVALUATION

Instructions: Mark your answers to the following questions with a black pen on the "Evaluation" section of your FasTrax® answer sheet provided with this course. You should not return this sheet. Please use the scale below to rate the following statements:

A   Agree Strongly   C   Disagree Somewhat
B   Agree Somewhat   D   Disagree Strongly

The course content met the following education objectives:

1. Discusses the responsibilities, attitudes, and skills needed to become an effective nurse supervisor.

2. Recognizes ways to accomplish unit and health care facility goals by working through others, and ways to build good human relations.

3. Identifies good communication skills, and how you can use these skills to maintain good staff relations.

4. Recognizes guidelines for directing staff and planning and conducting effective meetings.

5. Identifies ways to build cooperation and teamwork among nursing staff.

6. Recognizes ways to improve and maintain good client relations.

7. Identifies ways to organize and plan activities in your nursing unit.

8. Identifies ways you can employ time management techniques to increase your effectiveness as a nurse supervisor.

9. Discusses ways to coordinate and support team efforts.

10. Identifies skills needed for interviewing and orienting new nurses to your workplace.

11. Recognizes the nurse supervisor's function in training nursing staff.

12. Identifies appropriate methods for conducting performance appraisals.

13. Recognizes the steps to disciplining staff and procedures that should be used for dealing with grievances.

14. The content of this course was relevant to the objectives.

15. This offering met my professional education needs.

16. The objectives met the overall purpose/goal of the course.

17. The course was generally well written and the subject matter explained thoroughly. (If no please explain on the back of the FasTrax instruction sheet.)

18. The content of this course was appropriate for home study.

19. The final examination was well written and at an appropriate level for the content of the course.

Please complete the following research questions in order to help us better meet your educational needs. Pick the ONE answer which is most appropriate.

20. What nursing shift do you most commonly work?

    A. Morning Shift (Any shift starting after 3:00am or before 11:00am)

    B. Day/Afternoon Shift (Any shift starting after 11:00am or before 7:00pm)

    C. Night Shift (Any shift starting after 7:00pm or before 3:00am)

    D. I work rotating shifts

21. What was the SINGLE most important reason you chose this course?

    A. Low Price

    B. New or Newly revised course

    C. High interest/Required course topic

    D. Number of Contact Hours Needed

22. Where do you work? (If your place of employment is not listed below, please leave this question blank.)

    A. Hospital

    B. Medical Clinic/Group Practice/ HMO/Office setting

    C. Long Term Care/Rehabilitation Facility/Nursing Home

    D. Home Health Care Agency

23. Which field do you specialize in?

    A. Medical/Surgical

    B. Geriatrics

    C. Pediatrics/Neonatal

    D. Other

24. For your last renewal, how many months BEFORE your license expiration date did you order your course materials?

    A. 1–3 months

    B. 4–6 months

    C. 7–12 months

    D. Greater than 12 months

25. **PLEASE LOG YOUR STUDY HOURS WITH SUBMISSION OF YOUR FINAL EXAM.** Please choose which best represents the total study hours it took to complete this 30 hour course.

    A. less than 25 hours

    B. 25–28 hours

    C. 29–32 hours

    D. greater than 32 hours

CONTENTS

PRETEST

Begin by taking the pretest. Compare your answers on the pretest to the answer key (located in the back of the book). Circle those test items that you missed. The pretest answer key indicates the course chapters where the content of that question is discussed.

Next, read each chapter. Focus special attention on the chapters where you made incorrect answer choices. Exam questions are provided at the end of each chapter so that you can assess your progress and understanding of the material.

1. What increases when nurses in supervisory positions project decisiveness, confidence, and authority to their staff?

    a. anger and hostility

    b. security and productivity

    c. absences and complaints

    d. willingness to work extra shifts

2. Besides increasing work effectiveness, what happens when staff members are taught basic problem-solving skills?

    a. increased promotions

    b. decreased staff co-dependency

    c. reduced on-the-job stress

    d. increased delegation of duties

3. What helps staff nurses feel "in" on things?

    a. relaxed dress codes

    b. weekly staff meetings

    c. a monthly written report

    d. a unit suggestion box

4. What helps create a sense of self-worth among staff members?

    a. unloading boring or routine tasks on others

    b. performing tasks until they are experts

    c. giving directions to others

    d. having authority delegated to them

5. In what kind of working environment do most staff members gain greater personal satisfaction?

    a. authoritarian

    b. permissive

    c. structured

    d. democratic

6. Who needs to know patient/client assignment procedures and unit layout?

    a. a nurse on her first day of work

    b. patient families

    c. attending physicians

    d. housekeeping staff

7. When should a supervisor arrange practice and feedback for a skill deficiency?

    a. if the staff is new and inexperienced

    b. when the skill is new

    c. if staff members once had the skill but lost it

    d. when the skill is psychomotor

8. What helps health care facilities provide frank and constructive feedback to their staff?

    a. annual reports

    b. time management consultants

    c. performance appraisals

    d. HMO/PPO analyses

9. A perceptual filter is

    a. "how we view ourselves and others."

    b. "the way in which each of us distorts messages."

    c. "how people filter out negative statements."

    d. "the way environment influences our perception."

10. When people are afraid of unfavorable reactions, what are they likely to do?

    a. become quiet and unassertive

    b. transfer from job to job

    c. block their reception of feedback

    d. use poor speaking techniques

11. What type of communication is characterized by interaction?

    a. two-way communication

    b. democratic communication

    c. one-way communication

    d. internal communication

12. What acronym should you use to help you remember how to plan meetings?

    a. The Four Ws

    b. PAWS

    c. PLR

    d. FAST

13. Horizontal cooperation refers to your relationships with your

    a. peers.

    b. supervisors.

    c. subordinates.

    d. workers of the same sex.

14. What is most effective when it is solicited, well-timed, and checked for clear communication?

    a. delegation

    b. feedback

    c. team leading

    d. evaluations

15. Who is known for working together and encouraging active participation of all members?

    a. team leaders

    b. group members

    c. staff members

    d. unit leaders

16. Counseling is the method that should be used in addressing _____ problems.

    a. training

    b. morale

    c. performance

    d. disciplinary

17. Checking your resources is the first step in

    a. creating a weekly or a daily job plan.

    b. evaluating staff performance.

    c. planning a disciplinary action.

    d. responding to a grievance.

18. What do the rigid rules and policies of health care facilities sometimes cause?

    a. poor patient care

    b. barriers to communication

    c. increased liability for the staff

    d. inappropriate concern about asepsis

INTRODUCTION

Today's health care metamorphosis requires nurses to remaining open-minded and fluid in their response to change. To triumph over the challenges of change, nurses must strengthen their people skills. Nurses are now called upon to be coordinators and integrators of the delivery of client care. They are also surrendering many duties to health care partners under their supervision. Staff nurses, who in the past have only been responsible for managing the care of clients, are now being called on to guide and direct the work of others. Experienced nurse supervisors say, the biggest challenges they face daily arise from their interactions with clients, coworkers, and other health care professionals. This all adds up to a need for all nurses to increase their people skills.

People skills have always been part of the skills needed to "supervise." *Supervision* has been referred to as "the art of applying the science of behavioral technology." The essential ideas in this statement are as follows:

- Everyone who applies behavioral principles to their work is a supervisor.

- The application of behavioral principles is an art, not an exact process.

Because every successful nurse practices supervisory skills, they are not only important to nurses aspiring to be department or unit managers, but also to nurses who provide direct client care and direct unlicensed personnel.

Communication is the central skill around which all the other supervisory skills are dependent. Without the skills to effectively communicate ideas, directions, and feelings, a supervisor has never been seen as successful. Based on this, a significant portion of *Supervisory Skills for Nurses* is dedicated to communication skills. These skills include talking with peers, clients, and supervisors; preparing written correspondence; and planning and leading meetings.

Teamwork, or collaboration with others, is another ability that is fundamental to client care. Nurses have intuitively understood this for years. When professionals on teams are given more responsibility and authority, the results are better quality care, more efficiency, and, most important, **more professional satisfaction.**

Supervisory Skills for Nurses covers many personal skills that impact a nurse's job satisfaction. Skills such as time management, delegation, prioritizing, and planning tasks are often underemployed, causing job frustration. Techniques to help improve these skills are provided.

Most supervisors find assessing and directing the work of others to be a responsibility that requires many interpersonal skills. These skills include communication (talking, listening, and writing), planning, delegating, and reinforcing. The course reviews the administration of performance appraisals. It also recommends steps to take to address grievances or complaints.

Supervisory Skills for Nurses addresses a wide range of skills. The best way to learn interpersonal skills is through practice. Practice is provided throughout this course via a number of activities.

Every facility or health care organization will have its own policies and procedures. *Supervisory Skills for Nurses* has been designed to help participants implement their organization's policies and procedures. Many of the chapter activities are designed to help participants practice skills within their organization's structure and regulations.

Supervisory Skills for Nurses is focused on providing the "big picture" of the skills needed to be a successful supervisor. The course is not intended to encompass all the components of supervision. Rather, it aims to prepare participants for advancement to positions that require them to provide increased guidance to others. *Supervisory Skills for Nurses* will help participants refine their people skills—an achievement most nurses regard as an integral part of their professional development.

CHAPTER 1

THE ROLE OF THE NURSE SUPERVISOR

INTRODUCTION

Nursing roles have evolved along with major changes in health care. Today's health care environment demands that all nurses have the skills to supervise unlicensed assistive personnel (UAPs), and the skills to act as patient-care managers. In recent years nurses have begun to spend much more time supervising others (Fisher, 1996). Whether you are supervising UAPs or have been recently promoted to supervise other nurses, you are no longer looking at work as a non-supervisory employee. You have begun to view your job, and many people you work beside, through the eyes of a nurse supervisor.

CHAPTER OBJECTIVE

After studying this chapter, you will be able to recognize the responsibilities, attitudes, and skills needed to become an effective nurse supervisor.

LEARNING OBJECTIVES

Upon completion of this chapter, you will be able to:

1. Differentiate the responsibilities and attitudes of non-supervisory staff, and the responsibilities and attitudes of nurse in the role of supervisor.

2. Identify knowledge, skills, and attitudes you will need to develop to become an effective nurse supervisor.

3. Identify knowledge, skills, and attitudes you already have that will help you to be effective as a supervisor.

LESSON CONTENT

This chapter introduces you to the role of the nurse as a supervisor, and describes how it is different from non-supervisory roles. Within this chapter you will discover some of the ways responsibilities, relationships, and attitudes change for nurses in the supervisory position. You will learn about some of the skills you need, and the valuable knowledge, skills, and experience you already have that make your job as a supervisor easier.

Most nurses already have many of the skills they need to become supervisors. As you read the following text, take a moment to complete the activities. They will give you a good idea of what you already know how to do, and what you still need to learn. As you complete each activity, don't limit your thinking to what you do at work. Think about the knowledge, skills, and experience you have acquired through roles other than that of a nurse such as mother, father, sister, brother, or friend and through activities such as PTA, church groups, volunteer work, political organizations, and other groups to which you belong.

ADJUSTMENTS IN RESPONSIBILITIES

When you are not in a supervisory role, your interactions are primarily with your co-workers, patients, families, doctors, and your nursing unit's coordinators and managers. In the non-supervisory role, you are responsible for your own work, your own behavior, and your own job performance. In the nurse supervisor role, you are still responsible for your own work, your own behavior, and your own job performance. In addition, your work, your behavior, and your job performance are all tied in with the work, behavior, and job performance of the staff whom you supervise. Their success is your success.

Nursing supervisory responsibilities fall into four basic categories:

- Communicating
- Working Through People
- Organizing and Planning
- Managing

Communicating

In the role of nurse supervisor, you are responsible for maintaining good employee relations and good public relations. As a supervisor, you interact more closely with management and the public. For example, you may be called upon to intercede when patients, patient families, or physicians have a complaint concerning your health care facility's policies or procedures. The ability to communicate well both orally and in writing is crucial to your success as a nurse supervisor. Good listening skills and the ability to provide constructive feedback are also essential elements.

ACTIVITY

On the following self-assessment chart (and on the charts that appear throughout this chapter), check the appropriate column for each of the knowledge or skill statements. Be as honest with yourself as you can. (This is for your information only!) Repeat this activity wherever the self-assessment charts appear in this chapter. Use the completed charts to plan your professional development and your work on this course.

SELF-ASSESSMENT CHART	ALWAYS	MOST OF THE TIME	SOMETIMES	NEVER
HUMAN RELATIONS				
I like to build good relationships with others.				
I have a positive attitude.				
I am sensitive to the feelings of others.				
I am patient with the mistakes of others.				
I am not afraid to admit my own mistakes.				
I understand that my moods affect others.				
I have a good sense of humor.				
I have confidence in my own ability.				
I can usually remain positive under stress.				
I treat people equally regardless of sex, culture, religion, age, or educational background.				
COMMUNICATIONS				
I am a good listener.				
I can write clearly and concisely.				
I speak well in front of others.				
I give clear, straightforward verbal directions.				
I give tactful and constructive feedback.				
I am courteous and helpful on the phone.				
I communicate well with nurse supervisors.				
I communicate well with peers.				
I am a good teacher.				
I ask questions when I need help.				

Working Through People

Few, if any, nurse supervisors can accomplish unit goals without the efforts of others. An effective supervisor assigns tasks and responsibilities to help everyone contribute to the overall productivity of the unit. An effective nurse supervisor also encourages staff members to pool their ideas and work together toward common goals.

SELF-ASSESSMENT CHART	ALWAYS	MOST OF THE TIME	SOMETIMES	NEVER
WORKING THROUGH PEOPLE				
I enjoy working with others toward a common goal.				
I invite the suggestions and ideas of others.				
I understand that each individual has unique abilities.				
I often give people positive reinforcement.				
I enjoy helping others develop their skills.				
I like sharing credit with others.				
I am able to stimulate others to be motivated.				
I am comfortable assigning responsibilities to others.				

Organizing and Planning

Organizing and planning play a critical role in the nurse supervisor's job. Supervisors work through others to accomplish unit goals. Nurse supervisors must know their unit's resources, assess patient assignments, and establish work priorities. They then must match staff and resources to jobs.

SELF-ASSESSMENT CHART	ALWAYS	MOST OF THE TIME	SOMETIMES	NEVER
ORGANIZING/PLANNING SKILLS				
I am a very organized person.				
I make a plan for each day.				
I accomplish most of what I plan to do each day.				
It is easy for me to keep my priorities in order.				
It is easy for me to find what I need in my work space.				
I work at a pace I find comfortable.				
My daily schedule is flexible enough to accommodate emergencies.				
I like to involve others in the planning process.				

Managing

Some nurse supervisors are responsible for developing and managing unit activities. Nurse supervisors may be called upon to:

- Interview, hire, and orient new staff.
- Recognize training needs and provide on-the-job training.
- Communicate unit and staff needs to management.
- Communicate patient, family, and sometimes physician needs to management.
- Evaluate professional and nonprofessional staff job performance.
- Evaluate staffing needs on a daily basis.
- Provide safe staffing and safe working conditions.

SELF-ASSESSMENT CHART	ALWAYS	MOST OF THE TIME	SOMETIMES	NEVER
MANAGING				
I understand my job very well.				
I understand the health care facility and unit goals.				
I have a good knowledge of the health care facility policies in regard to personnel management functions.				
I have a good knowledge of the health care facility policies in regard to safety issues.				
I have good knowledge of laws concerning patient records and charting.				
I am comfortable with evaluating the performance of my staff.				
I like teaching people how to do something new.				
I find it easy to see a situation from another's point of view.				
I am good about taking notes during meetings.				
My filing systems are logical and easy to use.				
I am aware of the impact personal problems can have on an individual's work.				

ADJUSTMENTS IN RELATIONSHIPS

When you assume your supervisory responsibilities, your relationships with other nurses will be different than when you were in a non-supervisory role. You may even be promoted, and placed in charge of nurses who were formerly your co-workers. You may end up forming peer relationships with people who were formerly your supervisors. If this is the case, the very nature of your interactions with co-workers and other supervisors will change to accommodate your new position.

Relationships with Non-supervisory Staff

You can expect your relationships with previous nurse co-workers to change when you are promoted above their level of authority. They will see you as management, even if you are not their direct supervisor. It is essential for you to recognize and prepare yourself for the kind of changes that will occur so that you can take steps to smooth the adjustment process.

Staff Expectations

As a staff member, you join your co-workers in following the instructions of your supervisors. You may rely on these people to inspire you to achieve unit goals. You depend on your supervisors to interpret management's directives and to intercede on your behalf. You may consult your supervisor when you experience problems on the job. And, you count on your supervisors to provide you with formal and informal feedback on your job performance.

When you work in a supervisory position, your staff will expect you to

Lead. Your staff will expect you to take charge, make decisions, and provide them with assignments.

Motivate. Your staff will expect you to inspire them, provide direction, and keep up morale.

Mediate. Your staff will expect you to interpret management directives and approach management with their concerns.

Advise and Counsel. Your staff will expect you to listen to their concerns and provide them with advice.

Evaluate. Your staff will rely on you to provide them with regular feedback on their performance.

Making Changes

Whether you are in a new environment or a familiar environment, you probably will see things you would like to change when you take a new position. You may have several good ideas for improving operations and staff effectiveness. These ideas, and your enthusiasm for your new job, may tempt you to make sweeping changes. Before you make changes though, stop and think. What your staff needs from you right now is a sense of stability. During the period of transition, reassure them that you do not intend to make alterations in personnel, equipment, or procedures in the immediate future. If you allow everyone to adjust gradually without major disruptions, your staff will be more receptive and less resentful when you do make changes (Tappen, 1995).

Friendships with Former Co-Workers

One of the important issues you may confront in a new position is handling friendships with other nurses you now supervise. This can be a tricky situation and must be treated carefully. Clearly, you don't want to give up your friendships just because you've been promoted. However, you also can't allow your friendships to influence your ability to treat all staff fairly and objectively. Even the appearance of favoritism can be extremely destructive to the atmosphere of cooperation you are trying to create. The key to good supervision is to establish and maintain open and healthy relationships with all your staff.

Voice of Authority

As a staff nurse, you listen to and may even join your co-workers in expressing their feelings about patient assignments, superiors, and other nurse co-workers. Nurse co-workers may ask your opinion about problems they are having on and off the job. This sharing of personal information can sometimes lead to awkward situations, even when you and the other staff member are functioning in similar positions. However, it is especially precarious to share personal information when you are acting as the other person's supervisor. You now may represent management to previous co-workers and your voice has the authority of "the boss" behind it. Casual comments and advice will have a greater impact than they did before you became the other staff member's supervisor. Be careful about what you say and how you say it. Also, remember never to say or write anything you don't wish to hear about later. Words have a way of coming back to haunt you.

Relationships with Upper Management

Because you are in a new position and your superiors may not know you in your new role, it is particularly important for you to take time to build relationships of trust and mutual respect.

Discussed below are some ways you can build such relationships.

Demonstrate your ability to communicate clearly, honestly, and on a regular basis. Your superiors will feel more secure if they know what is going on and where you stand. Your staff will feel more secure when they know you can represent them with upper management.

Demonstrate that you understand the importance of achieving health care facility and unit goals in a timely manner. Let your superiors know that you understand the importance of time by being on time for work, making sure your unit's work is completed, being prepared for meetings, and submitting reports on time. Let them know that you understand the missions and goals of the health care facility and the nursing department and how they relate to your unit's activities.

Ask for help when needed during the transition period after a promotion. Your boss will respect you for your willingness to acknowledge your limits and, consequently you will be less likely to make mistakes.

When you supervise others, you help build the morale of the staff you supervise, so they will work effectively and maintain high quality patient care. At the same time, it is important to support management and implement the goals they have set for the unit. At times, you will have to absorb pressure from both those you supervise and your superiors. If you have taken the time to build good relationships with both sides, you will find it easier to maintain your balance and perspective in this situation.

ADJUSTMENTS IN ATTITUDES

Attitude is your mental outlook. It is the way you look at and feel about things. Your attitude as a nurse supervisor sets the tone of your relationships with all those with whom you work. Having a positive attitude toward the job, your own supervisor, and your staff goes a long way in securing the trust, respect, and willing cooperation that you need to perform your job effectively.

The Power of a Positive Attitude

There is a direct relationship between your attitude and the attitude of those you supervise. These staff members will look to you for cues as to how they should feel and act. Approaching your job in a tentative or negative fashion, consistently being late to work, or complaining about your job will have a negative impact on the attitudes and behavior of other staff members. On the other hand, if you are positive and upbeat about your job, if you begin each workday energetically, if you handle mistakes calmly, and if you accept minor setbacks with good humor, you will communicate that you accept responsibilities enthusiastically. Other staff will respond in positive ways that enhance cooperation and high-quality patient care. Through your attitude you gain the power to affect the way the staff you supervise and your superiors see you. You influence their behavior, and gain their trust and respect.

Projecting a Stronger Image

When you are not acting in the role of supervisor, you may not have many opportunities to exercise your leadership skills because others are in charge and make many of the major decisions. You usually interact with others in the style of an employee rather than in the style of a supervisor. When you begin to act as a supervisor, you need to modify your work style to include more leadership qualities.

Staff members like to work for a supervisor who is energetic, motivated, and keeps them moving in the right direction. Workers feel more secure and tend to produce more when they are part of a cohesive group led by an individual who establishes structure and guidelines. Some of the qualities staff members look for in a strong leader includes the following.

Confidence. You may not have as much confidence as you would like when you first step into the shoes of a supervisor, but becoming a nurse supervisor is an excellent way to practice your leadership skills and to increase your level of self-confidence.

Decisiveness. It is important to everyone that you demonstrate an ability to make decisions. Although those you supervise will offer ideas and suggestions, and be actively involved in team efforts, someone needs to bring it all together and make the final decisions—and that person is you!

Authority. Be sensitive about the way you exercise your authority. Keep in mind that you don't have to be a highly verbal extrovert to demonstrate authority. Quiet, sensitive people with inner strength are often excellent supervisors.

Ability to Delegate. A nurse supervisor needs to distribute tasks fairly and evenly, drawing upon the special talents of each individual, and, when appropriate, rotating responsibilities among various staff members.

Professional Appearance. The way you dress reflects the way you think of yourself and affects the image you project to others. If you are sloppily dressed, people will tend to believe that you conduct your work in a sloppy fashion. A neat appearance, on the other hand, gives the impression that you are organized and in control. It is usually better to dress up than to dress down when you step into a management position, but don't overdo it! The essential thing to remember is that the impression you create is always important.

Sense of Humor. You may be surprised at how responsive people can be when authority is balanced with the ability to laugh at oneself and at the sometimes amusing situations occur in our everyday work. It effectively demonstrates an ability to take obstacles in stride and reduces stress. As with any of the qualities mentioned, humor needs to be used appropriately and with sensitivity.

WHAT BEING A GOOD NURSE SUPERVISOR CAN DO FOR YOU

Your move into a new position or just improving the skills you use with the current staff you supervise, offers you a chance to grow professionally and personally. As you increase the staff you supervise, you increase your earning potential and position yourself for future promotions. Supervision can provide an opportunity to try out and develop your existing leadership, human relations, and communications skills; to build and maintain mutually rewarding relationships; and to experience the benefits of working through a team of staff members. Finally, stepping into the role of nurse supervisor and practicing nurse supervisory skills can build your self-confidence and increase your self-esteem.

SUPPLEMENTAL ACTIVITIES

1. After you've completed all the self-assessments in this Chapter, make an appointment with your boss/supervisor and show him/her the assessments. Explain your own opinions and ask your supervisor for opinions. Take notes about your boss/supervisor's opinions. Make an appointment for another assessment in six months and compare the results.

2. Ask your boss/supervisor to explore with you one or all of the following questions.

   a. What is a "typical day" in the life of a supervisor?

   b. What are the characteristics and principles

of good supervision?

c. How did you, as a nurse supervisor handle relationships with co-workers just after promotion?

d. What are the positive and negative aspects of being a supervisor?

e. How did you handle stress?

3. Think of a successful nurse supervisor whom you respect. Compare this person's performance to the list of qualities in "Projecting a Stronger Image," above, and note which ones the supervisor displays.

EXAM QUESTIONS

CHAPTER 1
Questions 1–4

1. Janet is in an interview with her boss to discuss the possibility of becoming a supervisor. Which of the statements made by Janet would indicate she already has some of the skills that will make her an effective nurse supervisor?

   a. "I have the ability to get my way most of the time."

   b. "When I am in a position of authority I don't kid around."

   c. "I like to listen to people's views on things."

   d. "I let people figure things out for themselves."

2. How should your promotion to a supervisory position affect your comments or advice to others at work?

   a. You should keep your advice to yourself.

   b. Advice should be given out more often.

   c. You must exercise more care in your comments and advice.

   d. There should be no change in your comments or advice.

3. You have been Beth and Marisa's supervisor for the past two years. Beth is a close friend. Marisa is a good worker, but not a friend. Both nurses handed in requests on the same day for a one week vacation from July 1–7. If your unit is to maintain adequate staffing, only one of them can be gone during this week. How should you handle the situation?

   a. Explain the situation and see if one will volunteer to change her plans. If neither will volunteer, tell them to work it out and get back to you.

   b. Turn the decision over to your supervisor so that no one will think you are playing favorites.

   c. Give the vacation to the non-friend so that no one will think you are playing favorites.

   d. Try to find replacements for both. Reject both requests if you can't find replacements.

4. In order to make staff feel more secure and productive, nurses in supervisory positions should be

   a. decisive, confident, and authoritative.

   b. extroverted, honest, and sensitive.

   c. relaxed, amiable, and flexible.

   d. authoritative, rigid, and strong.

CHAPTER 2

UNDERSTANDING HUMAN BEHAVIOR

INTRODUCTION

From the moment you step into a supervisory role, you begin working through others to accomplish unit and health care facility goals. Although your technical skills will be important in teaching and directing staff, you soon will discover that your technical abilities are not nearly as important as your human relation skills.

Good human relations for nurse supervisors are more than a matter of friendly and courteous behavior. Human relations also include

- generating loyalty, trust, and respect.
- building healthy working relationships.
- orienting staff to the expectation of goal achievement and quality workmanship.
- balancing individual needs with health care facility goals.
- supporting staff efforts to resolve conflicts.
- responding constructively to frustrations.

Building good human relations on the job is difficult if you don't understand human behavior and the factors that affect relationships. Human behavior is influenced by five important factors, each presented in separate parts of this chapter. They are

- motivational factors;
- human values;
- organizational norms;
- selective perception; and
- stress.

When you understand these factors and how they influence staff behavior, you are better able to inspire the people in your unit.

CHAPTER OBJECTIVE

After studying this chapter you will be able to recognize ways to accomplish unit and health care facility goals by working through others, and ways to build good human relations.

LEARNING OBJECTIVES

Upon completion of this chapter, you will be able to:

1. Indicate the type of skills most important in teaching and directing staff.

2. Recognize three of the five factors that influence human behavior.

3. Identify the human behavior factors that affect what people want from their work, and how they perform at work.

4. Recognize the working condition staff nurses rank highest.

5. Identify how these human behavior factors affect supervision.

6. Recognize appropriate ways of responding to work situations, based upon an understanding of these human behavior facts.

7. Select the correct definition for two of the common forms of selective perception.

8. Identify the advantages of a democratic working environment.

9. Identify factors that affect worker response to on-the-job stress and how a nurse supervisor can reduce stress.

LESSON CONTENT

People work for a variety of reasons. Some people work for basic survival needs, such as paying for food and a place to live, while others are seeking job or financial security. Some work for status, personal fulfillment, or to satisfy even deeper needs. What is important for one person may be unimportant to another.

YOUR MOTIVATIONS

What is important to you?

ACTIVITY

What do you want from your job? Look at the list below. Place a "1" before the most important item to you, "2" before the second most important item, and so on.

_____ Job security

_____ Tactful disciplining

_____ Good wages

_____ Feeling "in" on things

_____ Full appreciation for work done

_____ Sympathetic understanding of personal problems

_____ Good working conditions

_____ Interesting work

_____ Management loyalty to workers

_____ Promotion and growth with company

In hundreds of opinion polls conducted in both government and industry, pay ranked fifth in the order of preference. Does this surprise you? If pay isn't the most important thing employees want from their job, what is?

Several studies were designed to find out what supervisors thought workers wanted from their jobs, supervisors were asked to rank the same list you just did. The workers also ranked the items. The results for both groups are shown in the table on the next page.

As you can see, what supervisors thought workers wanted from a job and what workers said they wanted were very different. Supervisors believed workers wanted

*   good wages first.

*   job security second.

*   promotion third.

The workers said they wanted

*   full appreciation for work done first.

*   feeling "in" on things second.

*   sympathetic understanding of personal problems, third.

When staff members want one thing and a nurse supervisor thinks they want something else, the result can be dissatisfaction on both sides. The nurse supervisor encourages staff with incentives that don't match the staff's needs.

MEETING STAFF NEEDS

Each member of your nursing staff has a different set of needs and priorities. As a nurse supervisor, you'll discover the needs and priorities of the members of your staff over

Priority Ranking of Items	What Supervisors Thought Workers Wanted from Their Jobs	What Workers Said They Wanted from Their Jobs
1	Good wages	Full appreciation for work done
2	Job security	Feeling "in" on things
3	Promotion and growth with company	Sympathetic understanding of personal problems
4	Good working conditions	Job security
5	Interesting work	Good wages
6	Management loyalty to workers	Interesting work
7	Tactful disciplining	Promotion and growth with company
8	Full appreciation for work done	Management loyalty to workers
9	Sympathetic understanding of personal problems	Good working conditions
10	Feeling "in" on things	Tactful disciplining

time, through casual conversations, formal evaluations, and other work interactions. Once you know what motivates your staff, you can respond to these needs accordingly.

PROVIDING A MOTIVATIONAL ENVIRONMENT

Providing a motivational environment is the key to increasing organizational effectiveness. As a nurse supervisor, you'll need to strike a balance between the health care facility's needs and the staff's needs. This means considering the following

- the kind of health care being provided.

- the needs and characteristics of your staff members.

- your own needs and characteristics.

Based on what you learn about these three elements, you can build a working environment that best suits the situation in which you find yourself.

One way of looking at working environments is to divide them into three basic types: Structured, permissive, and democratic. The table that follows summarizes the characteristics of each system and presents some of the advantages and disadvantages of each.

TABLE OF WORKING ENVIRONMENTS		
TYPE OF ENVIRONMENT	ADVANTAGES	DISADVANTAGES
STRUCTURED		
Nurse supervisor maintains tight, restrictive control; sets goals and standards; expects staff to follow directions.	Works well for hazardous jobs and jobs with high-level safety requirements and for technical jobs that require high precision.	Will not meet the needs of staff members who need to feel "in" on things.
	Close supervision minimizes injuries and ensures that precision standards are met.	Experienced staff members may feel oppressed.
	Structure and close supervision provides security to insecure staff members.	Discourages creativity and independent thinking.
PERMISSIVE		
Nurse supervisor provides little or no leadership, few guidelines or restrictions, and little encouragement or feedback.	Atmosphere is relaxed and easygoing. Staff members can determine their own working style.	Inexperienced staff members with little self-discipline may lose the desire to succeed without goals, direction, and encouragement.
DEMOCRATIC		
Nurse supervisor involves the entire staff in planning and goal setting. Nurse supervisor is part of the group while retaining a leadership role.	Most staff members gain greater personal satisfaction. Encourages team achievement and individual creativity.	Requires sensitivity and experience. Inexperienced staff members may prefer a more structured environment until they feel more sure of themselves.

In a health care environment, many factors determine which management style works best in a given job, including:

- Which style you are most comfortable with as nurse supervisor.
- Whether you are working with experienced nursing staff who work well on their own, or with new nurses who need more guidance and direction.
- Whether the job requires close supervision for safety or quality's sake.
- Whether high-quality care can be maintained by peer double checks rather than direct supervision by a supervisor.

Some nurse supervisors combine a structured approach with a democratic approach. Others may create a working environment that includes features of all three basic types.

As a new nurse supervisor, it's a good idea to observe the unit's activities and people's personalities before drawing any conclusions about the best type of environment. Remember that your assumptions about what motivates your staff are bound to influence your leadership style. The more effectively you adapt your leadership style to the requirements of your particular job, the needs of your staff, and to your own personality characteristics, the more effectively you will meet personal and health care facility goals.

ACTIVITY

1. On a separate piece of paper, list all of the jobs you've held, including the one you have now.

2. For each job, briefly describe the way you were supervised.

3. For each job, list what you liked and didn't like about how you were supervised.

4. Compare your comments to the Table of Working Environments. Match the jobs and your descriptions of how you were supervised to the styles in the table.

5. In your current job, you may have been supervised differently when you were first hired than you are now. If so, list the differences.

6. If you are not completely satisfied with the way you are supervised now, write a brief description of how you would like to be supervised.

HUMAN VALUES

We all operate on the basis of principles, standards, or qualities we consider worthwhile or important to our well-being. These principles, standards, and qualities are our values. We learn our values through a variety of sources: a family, schools, places of worship, contact and interaction with others at work and in the community, and so on.

Your Values

Values tell us and others what is important in life. Some typical values include

- belonging to a church, temple, or synagogue and to attending regularly.

- obtaining a college education.

- owning a late model sports utility vehicle.

- doing everything to the best of your ability.

- making sure no one steals from you.

- having others believe you are self-confident, even when you're feeling unsure.

- always telling the truth.

- being appreciated for your abilities, not how you look.

ACTIVITY

The list above may or may not reflect any of your own personal values. Think about your life at work, at home, with your friends and family. Write down four or five of your values—the things you believe are important in life. _____

_____

_____

_____

_____

Our values usually become apparent when we must choose between two of them.

Example

Jill began working as a staff nurse on a pediatric ward of a large metropolitan hospital. She valued feeling like a part of the group and started making friends among the other nurses. After a few days, Jill discovered that a number of her co-workers were feuding. The two groups tended to gossip about each other. She realized that another of her values was to stay away from nasty gossip.

Jill made a choice: she worked on friendships with the people not involved in the feud and remained polite but distant with the others until the feud ended.

RESPONDING TO THE EFFECTS OF HUMAN VALUES

It will be part of your job as nurse supervisor to weigh the impact of different values in various on-the-job situations. In some cases, you will need to help nurses resolve conflicts that can arise from a clash of values. In helping to resolve disagreements, it is important to assure each staff member that all their value systems are important.

If you can create an atmosphere that integrates various personalities and fosters respect for individual values, your staff will begin to value working for you and will be more willing to cooperate and compromise when it becomes necessary. Don't expect too much of yourself at first, though. Learning to spot other people's values and respond to them takes time.

ORGANIZATIONAL NORMS

Organizational norms also have an important role in influencing the way people behave at work. Organizational norms are standard, currently accepted methods of doing things in an organization. They are specific guides to conduct and provide a way for individuals to organize and structure their behavior (Sullivan, 1994).

Formal vs. Informal Norms

Norms can be formal or informal. Formal norms are backed up by written policies. Fire and safety procedures, sexual harassment policy, chain of command procedures, infection control procedures, and workday length are formal norms.

Most formal norms are easy to understand and we have no difficulty following them. Some of our more recently instituted formal norms, however, like prevention of sexual harassment, are not well understood by all and often ignored or taken lightly. It is the nurse supervisor's job to help staff become aware of behaviors that are inappropriate and the serious consequences of sexual harassment.

Other formal norms that are sometimes taken lightly with grave consequences are fire and safety codes, ergonomic program guidelines, medication checking procedures, and infection control procedures.

Formal norms are just the "tip of the iceberg." Most norms are informal, unwritten "agreements." Sometimes they exist even when the formal norms say they shouldn't. For instance, in most hospitals it is considered inappropriate to wear a low-cut blouse or uniform to work. Although the hospital may not have a rule that specifies this, most people choose to follow this unwritten "rule." Most of us are not consciously aware of the norms to which we conform.

Examples of informal norms in hospitals can include the following:

- Do not talk in a loud voice.
- Allow gurneys and wheelchairs on the elevators first.
- Offer help to visitors who look lost.
- Don't borrow co-workers' equipment without permission.
- Don't talk about your personal life in front of patients.
- Don't wear heavy make-up or cologne.

You can get a good indication of the norms present in your day-to-day work environment and how they influence your behavior and the behavior of others by taking a few minutes to do the following activity.

ACTIVITY

1. On a separate piece of paper, list the informal norms that seem to operate on your unit. List standards (written or unwritten), laws, etc., to which the health care facility work force appears to conform. They should represent things that actually happen.

Examples:

- Interviewers usually dress more formally on interview days.

- Doctors and nurses should not talk about social events in the unit corridor.

- Ethnic jokes or jokes about sexuality are not okay.

2. Make a list of norms (usually backed by policy) operating on your own unit.

Examples:

- Work schedules are posted.

- Staff nurses must get the nurse supervisor's approval before working overtime.

- The nurse supervisor makes sure that new nurses are introduced to the rest of the staff.

- We take pride in our helpfulness toward clients' families.

EFFECTS OF NORMS ON BEHAVIOR AT WORK

Conflicts and other difficulties can arise if you are not aware of the norms in effect in your department, unit, or agency. If you choose not to abide by these norms or if you don't understand how they interact with your values and the values of others, you can also have problems.

Norms and values can match up or clash with one another. For example, the hospital supports the value of equality by establishing specific nondiscriminatory procedures or norms for hiring and selection. In this case, hospital norms (nondiscriminatory standards) are in harmony with values. However, norms can also clash with values. In fact, norms may actually interfere with people's ability to obtain what they value, as demonstrated in the example that follows.

Example

Cheryl is a charge nurse in a psychiatric facility where street clothes are accepted dress code. Cheryl has a unique personal style. She likes unusual clothing and haircuts, and large "clunky" jewelry. Although she is considered well-groomed and appropriately dressed for her position, she attracts a certain amount of attention because of her unconventional appearance.

After a few months in her job, Cheryl notices that the nurse supervisors and staff in management tend to dress more formally and more conservatively than she does. She also notices that the people who say they want to be promoted tend to dress the same way—conservatively and less casually.

Cheryl faces a dilemma. She values the way she expresses herself through her clothing, *and* she wants to be promoted someday.

As you probably can see, there is no right or wrong to Cheryl's problem. Because her appearance is within the guidelines of the health care facility dress code, Cheryl cannot be required to change her appearance. She may be promoted without conforming to the norm. But, she recognizes that her best chances of promotion lie in not opposing the norm. Cheryl will have to decide whether it's more important to her to dress and look the way she wants, or to be promoted into the job she wants. She may be able to find a compromise that is comfortable for her.

RESPONDING TO THE EFFECTS OF ORGANIZATIONAL NORMS

When you are a supervisor, becoming aware of the norms that operate on your unit and in your health care facility helps you gain insight into accepted behaviors. This will allow you to make more informed decisions regarding your staff and their responsibilities. Informal norms are not always easy to see. You'll need to make a conscious effort to become aware of them.

The better you understand the values and norms of your unit's staff, the better you will be able to understand why your staff behaves the way they do, why they are or are not motivated, why they work hard, and why some may tend to avoid certain responsibilities (Sullivan, 1994). You can use such knowledge and awareness to solve existing problems; anticipate potential conflicts; and to modify norms, when appropriate, to support staff job functions.

SELECTIVE PERCEPTION

Perception refers to the way we interpret information we receive through our five senses—seeing, hearing, touching, tasting, and smelling—and relate that information to what we already know or believe. Selective perception occurs when we sense only part of what is presented to us. All humans use selective perception. This can work to our advantage, by simplifying our world and helping organize it into a reasonably stable, predictable place. However, selective perception can also cause us to ignore or distort information that contradicts our beliefs or values,

and to exaggerate information that is consistent with what we believe or value. When this occurs, we can hurt others, block communication and stifle creativity.

Using Selective Perception

Human perception is selective—that is, we sense only what we need or want to sense. If we didn't "filter out" most of the sensory information the world provides us with each day, we would not be able to get anything done. We would be overwhelmed. Instead, we pay close attention to some information, little attention to other information, and ignore or simply don't register other types of information.

Example

- Smokers tend not to see items dealing with the relationship between cancer and smoking.
- Anxious family members may focus on when they cannot visit rather than when they can visit.
- Hearing that the I.M. injection will sting rather than how it will ease the postoperative pain.
- Heavy drinkers tend to ignore information on alcoholism.

Selective perception is at work when you try to listen to a patient talk when the television is turned on. You learn to "tune out" the television.

Other examples of selective perception follow.

Some of the more common forms of selective perception are

- categorizing;
- stereotyping;
- halo effect; and
- projecting.

Each of these forms of selective perception will be discussed.

Categorizing

As human beings, we have the ability to classify information. We can arrange our thoughts and experiences into categories, and we can describe what we see by labeling it. In this course, for instance, we have categorized health care facility staff members into two groups: Those who supervise others and those who don't.

Categories help us

*   simplify our thinking.
*   rapidly identify related objects.
*   fit new information into what we already know.

However, categorization can also

*   distort our thinking processes (because we may not always base our categories on facts or rational criteria).
*   cause us to place events or people into inappropriate categories.

ACTIVITY

Two categories common to many work environments are "US" and "THEM." Sometimes staff members refer to themselves as "US" and to management as "THEM." Sometimes managers refer to themselves as "US" and to their staff as "THEM."

List the ways that the "US and THEM" categories distort your thinking about individuals.

Once you have categorized someone as one of **THEM,** you blind yourself to that person's individuality. In your viewpoint, **THEY** don't have the human qualities you do, and so you don't have to consider **THEIR** motivations or feelings.

The real risk in categorizing is once done, it is difficult to undo, even when new information contradicts your viewpoint. Prejudice is born and nourished by this kind of thinking.

Stereotyping

A stereotype is an oversimplified concept, opinion, or belief. You may be aware of some of the stereotypes that exist for mothers-in-law (**nosy, interfering**), for politicians (**corrupt, unethical**), for professors (**absent-minded**), or types of patients (**demanding, whining**). Many of us initially adopt stereotypical perceptions from our social groups and families. Then, as we encounter people in the groups we have stereotyped, we selectively look for evidence in their behaviors that support our adopted belief. In most cases the stereotype has little to no foundation in fact.

Like categorizing, stereotyping allows us to justify and rationalize our acceptance or rejection of a group of people or of an individual who is seen as a member of that group. Unlike categorizing, stereotyping makes assumptions about an individual's qualities or motivations based on that person's membership in a group.

ACTIVITY

List all the stereotypes you can think of for a nurse supervisor. Here are a few to get you started.

*   Cold
*   Overly ambitious
*   Critical
*   Perfectionist

The Halo Effect

The halo effect refers to a process in which your general impression about a person—positive or negative—determines your conclusions about the person's other specific traits. For example, if you determine that Robert Woods communicates well, and you decide that means he is also an excellent decision maker, creative thinker, and high producer, you are operating under the halo effect. Some nurse supervisors have been known to give good overall ratings to staff whose only known virtue was punctuality. Operating under the halo effect can result in some very poor decisions.

ACTIVITY

Think about your work situation for a moment. On a separate piece of paper, write down examples of how you, your co-workers, and your supervisor may be using the halo effect.

Projecting

Projection is the tendency to explain other people's behavior in terms of our own characteristics. For example, a nurse supervisor who does not have the ability to delegate might see others as having that same problem. A staff member worried about being laid off may see others as being more worried than they actually are about the same thing. Both the nurse supervisor and the staff member are projecting their own insecurities onto others.

Projection can blind us to the motivations, values, and feelings of others and can be a serious barrier to establishing healthy working relationships.

ACTIVITY

Think about your work situation again. Write down examples of how you, your co-workers, and your supervisor may project personal characteristics or feelings onto others.

IMPROVING INTERPERSONAL PERCEPTION

You will be a much better nurse supervisor if you start right now to increase your awareness of when and where you are using selective perception and of how it may be influencing your decisions about situations and people.

ACTIVITY

Review the lists you made of examples of categorizing, stereotyping, the halo effect, and projecting. On a separate piece of paper, write down specific ways in which these examples of selective perception might be affecting thinking and behavior. For example: Jane views Doug (a staff nurse) as 'most likely gay' because he is a male working in a job traditionally chosen by females. Therefore, when Jane makes patient assignments, she assigns Doug to older male patients. Jane is afraid younger male patients may feel uncomfortable having Doug take care of them.

In completing this activity or the earlier ones, did you find areas where selective perception was affecting your judgment? If you did, you have taken an important step toward changing your behavior. You need to evaluate new information carefully before making judgments, and stay alert to how the beliefs of your peers and family influence you. Then, you will be on your way to correcting stereotypes, and faulty perceptions, and minimize misjudgments in the future.

Did you suddenly understand the cause of some friction between co-workers that you've noticed? If you did, you're beginning to exercise another function of nurse supervisors—to help others see their selective perceptions and how those perceptions have influenced their working relationship.

ON-THE-JOB STRESS

Each day brings events that impact our behavior. When these events interfere with or complicate our efforts to reach our goals, we experience stress.

Research suggests that nursing is a highly stressful occupation. This is the reason for the high degree of "burn out" in nursing. Many of you may have already tried to learn ways to manage work stress early in your careers as a nurses. Although none of us manage to go through life without experiencing some degree of work stress, we can learn to keep its damaging side-effects to a minimum.

The Importance of Managing Stress

Your way of dealing with stress can affect your ability to enjoy life. Ignoring the impact of stress can result in ulcers, heart disease, high blood pressure, psychological illness, or cause relationship problems (Bradley, 1990). Making a positive effort to relieve the effects of stress can help you take your worries in stride and grow in the process.

The way you perceive and react to stress as a nurse supervisor will have a tremendous impact on your staff. Some of your staff may never have learned appropriate means for reducing stress or methods for solving problems. Chances are they will take their cues from you. If, in addition to serving as a positive example, you also take the time to teach your staff tools for managing their own stress, you will have increased dramatically the capacity you and your staff have for achieving organizational goals.

Sources of Stress

Individuals and groups experience stress both on and off the job. Stress can originate from external or internal sources.

External Sources

Stress can come from various sources outside ourselves. Listed below are some possible sources of stress.

- Work
- Illnesses of family or friends
- Problems with home or car
- Disagreements with family or friends

- Financial uncertainty
- Discipline problems with children
- Marital discord

Stress can even come from happy occasions such as weddings, births, recreational activities, or your promotion to supervising others. Even "happy stress" requires our energy and time and usually means we need to rest and recover.

Social pressures—restrictions and regulations society places on our behavior—can be particularly stressful. The organizational norms discussed earlier are a good example of social pressure. Stress can result when these organizational norms interfere with our achievement of goals and when we worry about what will happen if we ignore or break the "rules."

Internal Sources

Stress also can originate from within ourselves. Physical handicaps, illness, fatigue, and lack of needed skills can cause a tremendous amount of anxiety and threaten our ability to cope with day-to-day activities.

The feeling of having no control on the job is another internal source of stress. This stress is particularly common for nurses because there are frequently several unplanned events in a nurse's day (Douglas, 1996). Examples of these events include

- emergency admissions/walk-in patients in distress.
- patients who were stable taking a turn for the worse.
- inadequate staffing.
- being "floated" to another part of the hospital.
- having to wear personal pagers.
- frequent changes in technology and equipment.

Conflict

Conflict can originate internally or externally. Conflict can arise between individuals and groups or when an individual has to choose between two values or goals. Unresolved conflicts can cause such tension and inner turmoil that an individual's ability to adjust and cope is overtaxed.

ACTIVITY

1. List your internal sources of stress at work.

2. List your external sources of stress at work.

3. Write some ways you feel you can reduce both your internal and external sources of stress at work.

4. List your internal sources of stress at home.

5. List your external sources of stress at home.

6. Write down some ideas for reducing your internal and external stress at home.

Severity Of Stress

Stress is unavoidable. When you supervise other people, it is important to remember that it is not the existence of stress but the **severity** of the stress and the individual's tolerance for stress that decide if it is destructive. The severity of the stress is influenced by

- how long it lasts. The longer the stress lasts, the more severe it becomes.

- the number of stresses occurring at the same time.

- the cumulative effect of a series of minor stresses. Many stressful events in a row can strike an especially strong blow to an individual's ability to adapt.

- the importance of the need being obstructed by the stress. For example, if an important need such as security is threatened, the individual may suffer severe stress.

Perhaps one of the most important factors influencing the severity of stress is the individual's perception or evaluation of the stressful situation.

When you are supervising other people, you need to be aware of how different people will react differently to what you say.

REACTIONS TO STRESS

Individuals have different ways of coping with stress. Some are effective, others are not. Some of the more negative methods include

acting out—lashing out at others.

withdrawing—not talking to others and isolating yourself.

denying—ignoring or refusing to acknowledge the reality of an unpleasant situation.

projecting—thinking others have the same problems you have.

rationalizing—justifying what you do to soften your or others' disappointment at not reaching your goals.

compromising—settling for less than what you want to avoid conflict.

substance abuse—the use of drugs or alcohol to provide temporary relief from stress.

Almost all of us act out, withdraw, deny, project or rationalize from time to time. These coping strategies may help us feel better in the short run, but in the end they are not very helpful because they permit us to escape from rather than deal with the source of stress. In recent studies, nurses were found to be at particular risk for use and abuse of prescription medications, including controlled substances (Kozier, 1998).

Positive responses to stress include the following:

Enrolling in a self-help or support group. These groups are formed of people with a common concern, interest, or problem. By meeting on a regular basis, group members can share their experiences and their feelings, get advice and learn about their options. In support groups people learn that others also experience stressful reactions to their problems. Finding this out often helps people understand that they are not alone, or inadequate in coping with life. This knowledge helps them feel less stressed about their problems and their reactions to them.

Practicing meditation or self-hypnosis. Many easily learned meditation or self-hypnosis techniques allow people to quiet an overactive or frazzled mind. In this way, they give themselves a rest from thinking, planning, and worrying.

Scheduling "quiet times." Some people find that taking just an hour a day for completely "selfish" activity is all they need to counter the stress of their lives. New mothers spend the baby's morning nap time bathing and putting on makeup. Many people keep journals. Others need to sit and stare out a window, stroll on the beach, or listen to quiet music.

Engaging in regular physical exercise. Running, swimming, biking, or working out in an aerobics class helps many people "let off steam" at the end of a harrowing day. Even gentler forms of exercise, such as yoga, walking or modern dance, can take your mind off your worries for an hour or two.

Having a creative hobby. Painting, gardening, etc. As a nurse, you probably need to let the creative part of yourself out for a bit of exercise. You can find ideas for creative pursuits in a list of continuing education classes or recreation classes. Try basket making, sewing, sculpture, calligraphy, pottery—the list is endless.

ACTIVITY

List some of the more positive ways you have learned to respond to stress.

1. _____
2. _____
3. _____
4. _____
5. _____
6. _____
7. _____
8. _____
9. _____

WAYS TO REDUCE ON-THE-JOB STRESS

It is easy as a nurse supervisor to feel responsible for everything and everybody. You can trap yourself into spending a lot of time solving problems that your staff could solve themselves—possibly more effectively than you could—if given a chance. When you feel responsible for solving all the problems, you load an increasing amount of stress on yourself and leave yourself with little time to plan, organize, and supervise. In addition, you reduce the amount of control your staff feel over their situation and limit their personal growth.

One way you can help your staff reduce their own stress is to teach them to solve their own conflicts and problems. You can

- teach them basic problem-solving skills.

- provide tips for reducing stress.

- introduce them to hospital and community support resources.

Teach Basic Problem-Solving Skills

Having a systematic way of approaching problems is a great way to decrease anxiety and stress because it forces you to look at issues less emotionally. You can apply the same basic problem-solving steps (listed below) no matter what kind of problem you are dealing with.

Once you have learned to apply the problem-solving approach yourself, you can teach it to your staff so that they can resolve their concerns, problems, and conflicts either individually or through a group process. By teaching your staff to resolve their own problems, you will have shifted responsibility from yourself and will have reduced your stress level. And, you will have given your staff more control over their situation and provided an opportunity for them to grow.

1. **State the problem.** Write down as clearly as possible what you think defines the problem. If there is a conflict, get all parties involved in the conflict to agree before proceeding.

2. **Gather facts about the problem.** Write down when, where, and how the problem first occurred and who was involved. Decide how important it is in terms of money, time, effort, feelings, etc. Determine whether it will have a temporary or long-lasting impact. Determine the effect it is having on you. Decide whether it is a human relations issue that can blow out of proportion if you don't deal with it. Decide whether it is worth spending a lot of time and energy on.

3. **State the problem again.** Once you have looked at all the facts surrounding the problem, you may see it a different way. It may be more important or less important than you thought. It may not look the same at all.

4. **List the solutions you have already tried.** Write down every solution you have tried that didn't work. For each tried solution, write down why it didn't work. This process will help you take a careful look at what steps you actually have and haven't taken to resolve the situation.

5. **List solutions you haven't tried.** Look at alternative ways of handling the problem. Some of your ideas may seem silly at first, but list them anyway. If it is a human relations concern, look at your interactions with the other party or parties. Make sure you've considered the other person's motives, needs, and values. Consider communicating directly with the individual. Think about effective solutions you used in other situations and why they worked. Maybe they would work in this situation, too.

6. **List alternatives in terms of priority.** Think about which alternative solutions you think have the best chance of succeeding. Look at each solution and consider the benefits. Also, consider the risks and whether a given solution might create other problems. Organize your list with the best solution first, the next best solution second, and so on.

7. **Try out your best solution first.** Decide when and where you are going to try out the solution. Determine your approach. If it is an interpersonal issue, decide if it is appropriate to work it out privately or if others should be involved.

8. **Look at the results of your action.** Evaluate the results. Ask yourself if you got the desired result, or moved closer to a solution. If not, consider modifying the solution slightly and trying again. If it is a particularly difficult situation, you may need to try all of your solutions. Be sure to evaluate what happens each time and, if necessary, reevaluate the problem itself. If you still cannot resolve the problem, you may need to seek the assistance of your supervisor or someone else whose advice you trust.

Provide Tips for Reducing Stress

Most people already know ways to reduce stress, if they only remember to do them. When you are a nurse supervisor, you may need to remind yourself and your staff of the following.

1. **Learn to accept what you cannot change.** There are some things you can control and some you cannot. Concentrate on controlling the controllable items and refuse to worry about the others.

2. **Work off your frustration and anger.** When you're uptight, jog, walk, play tennis, or work in your garden or workshop at home. Whatever activity you choose, don't work at it so hard that it turns into an added source of stress.

3. **Balance work and recreation.** Everyone needs time off. Even you!

4. **Share your worries with someone you love, trust, or respect.** It almost always helps to talk to someone who cares about you and who listens. If necessary, seek the professional help of a psychologist, psychiatrist, or counselor.

5. **Take your mind off yourself.** Do something for others when you are upset. Get together with friends. Avoid using alcohol, drugs, or self-medication to escape your problems.

6. **Take one thing at a time.** When pressures on and off the job bear down on you from all sides, permit yourself to do one thing at a time. Ask yourself, "What's the best use of my time right now?" Accomplishing one thing will give you the energy to tackle the next, and ease the feeling of being overwhelmed.

Introduce Staff Members to Support Resources

Although one of your important jobs is to listen to the concerns of your staff, you will not have the time, energy, or the background for dealing with some of the more personal problems your staff may have. It is important for you to learn about the health care facility's resources such as employee counseling. Many organizations are offering help for employees who have drug, or alcohol abuse problems and will expect you to help identify and refer employees who need help.

SUPPLEMENTAL ACTIVITIES

1. Ask some of your co-workers to list in order of priority four or five things they want most from their jobs. See how they compare with your list.

2. Ask your nurse supervisor to list in order of priority four or five things staff members want most from their jobs (in your supervisor's opinion). See how this list compares with your list and those of your co-workers.

3. Find out what others see as norms for their organizations-whether or not they work for the health care facility.

4. Select a problem you are having either on or off the job. Solve it using the basic problem-solving steps.

5. Try out some new ways of reducing stress: walking, jogging, exercise, meditation, hobbies, or recreational activities. Make a chart of how much time you spend doing things that relax you and see if you can increase it.

CHAPTER 2
Questions 5–16

5. Understanding human behavior is important because it helps supervisors

   a. reprimand people in an effective way.

   b. understand the way people perform at work.

   c. categorize people effectively.

   d. give counseling to staff with family problems.

6. As a nurse who supervises others, developing _____ skills will help you most in achieving departmental and unit goals.

   a. technical

   b. human relations

   c. planning

   d. organizational

7. Supervisors should learn the organizational norms that are effective in their department

   a. so they can be written out as regulations.

   b. because being aware of them can help prevent conflicts.

   c. so they can be sure they always follow them.

   d. to "clean out" all norms so they don't affect productivity.

8. Three of the five important factors that influence human behavior are

   a. values, spirituality, and gender.

   b. race, age, and work ethic.

   c. values, stress, and motivation.

   d. leadership skills, prejudices, and motivation.

9. Factors that can affect whether stress is helpful or destructive to individuals in a work environment are

   a. whether the individuals are strong or weak types.

   b. how many co-workers also have stress.

   c. how many years the individual has been on the job.

   d. tolerance to stress and the severity of the stress.

10. What is one way supervisory nurses can help staff nurses reduce their on-the-job stress?

   a. Explain that people who overreact to stress seldom get promotions.

   b. Teach them basic problem-solving skills.

   c. Allow them time to go to counselors during work hours.

   d. Teach them to delegate duties that cause too much stress.

11. What is one advantage of a democratic working environment?

   a. Most staff members gain greater personal satisfaction.

   b. It is perfect for highly hazardous jobs.

   c. Staff can create their own work style.

   d. It is helpful for young and inexperienced employees.

12. "An oversimplified concept, opinion, or belief" is

   a. the halo effect.

   b. stereotyping.

   c. categorization.

   d. formalizing.

13. Which of the following work conditions would you expect staff nurses to rank highest?

   a. better than average pay

   b. high job security

   c. tactful disciplining

   d. full appreciation of work done

Questions 14–15 ask you to evaluate Linda's responses to the situation described below.

Linda supervises Michelle, a clinical lead nurse, and Tony, a staff nurse. One day, Tony comes to Linda with a complaint about Michelle. Tony said, "Michelle is too picky. She is not satisfied with anyone's client care and is always checking every little detail. It's getting really bad ... everyone feels they can never live up to her expectations."

Linda promises to look into the problem. When she meets with Michelle to hear her side of the dispute, Linda finds that Michelle is just as frustrated as Tony. "Tony and some of my nurses have this thing about getting their client care done quickly." Michelle said, "She wants all a.m. care done by 10 o'clock. I just don't think being fast is as important as being thorough."

14. The most likely basis of the conflict between Tony and Michelle is

   a. poor working conditions.

   b. a difference in values.

   c. lack of adequate supervision.

   d. an understaffed work unit.

15. What should Linda do about the conflict between Tony and Michelle?

   a. Nothing—these things tend to resolve themselves.

   b. Separate the two workers or re-assign them so they don't have to deal with each other anymore.

   c. Meet with Tony and Michelle to help them work out a solution themselves.

   d. Tell Tony and Michelle to each tend to their own work and quit criticizing each other.

16. What is the process in which a general impression about a person—positive or negative—determines your conclusion about the person's other specific traits?

   a. projection

   b. halo effect

   c. evaluating

   d. rationalizing

CHAPTER 3

BASIC COMMUNICATION SKILLS

INTRODUCTION

Your ability to communicate with others is crucial to your success as a nurse supervisor. In this chapter, you'll look at the factors that shape how you communicate and how you listen. You'll also learn what it takes to become a skillful communicator, how to listen effectively, and how to give feedback.

This chapter is organized into two parts.

Part One: What Is Communication?

Part Two: Listening Skills

CHAPTER OBJECTIVE

After studying this chapter, you will be able to identify good communication skills and how you can use these skills to maintain good staff relations.

LEARNING OBJECTIVES

Upon completion of this chapter, you will be able to:

1. Recognize how one acquires good communication skills.

2. Identify the definitions for communication, environment, feedback, and perceptual filters.

3. Recognize the role of cultural background in communications.

4. Recognize factors that influence communication and potential communication barriers.

5. Differentiate between positive and negative listening responses.

6. Identify the characteristics of one-way and two-way communication.

7. Recognize the disadvantages of one-way communication.

8. Indicate ways you can use good listening techniques.

PART ONE—WHAT IS COMMUNICATION?

The way you communicate is influenced by who you are. Who you are is determined in part by your experiences, background, biases, beliefs, and feelings—a combination unique to you. Our differences can add to the richness of our communications and our lives, or they can lead to communication breakdowns (Bradley, 1990). One of the duties of nurse supervisors and managers is to make sure such breakdowns are rare. Effective leaders are skillful communicators.

Most skillful communicators made a conscious decision to develop their skills. They found role models to watch, took courses (like this one), read books, evaluated their own performance under various conditions—and gradually came to be good listeners and clear speakers.

Good communication begins with the message sender. As sender, your function is to anticipate and remove barriers to communication. If communication breakdowns do occur, your job is to repair the rift.

Flexibility, rather than fixed rules, is the key. The following guidelines should give you a starting point.

DEFINING THE TERMS OF COMMUNICATION

This section uses several terms to talk about the process of communicating. You'll read more about each of these words or phrases. They are as follows:

Communication—the transfer of information. It is used to achieve a common understanding (not necessarily agreement) about a situation, object, or event. In oral transfers of information, communication occurs through the use of

- speech;
- facial expression;
- posture;
- tone, pitch, and volume of voice;
- timing and pace of speech; and
- eye contact.

Environment—the physical surroundings in which communication takes place. Environments can range from a quiet office to a noisy emergency room to a playing field in a park.

Feedback—a response to a message. When you give feedback, you relay your feelings about or understanding of a message you received. When you ask for feedback, you are checking to see whether your message was received as you intended.

Message—a piece of information. The message you intend to send may or may not be the message that is received; use feedback to check.

Perceptual filters—the ways in which each of us distorts messages. The negative consequence of our perceptual filters is balanced by feedback, which corrects the misunderstandings caused by our filters.

Receiver—a person who hears a message communicated by a sender.

Sender—a person who relays a message to a receiver. The sender and receiver roles reverse many times during a given exchange.

One-Way vs. Two-Way Communication

Two-way communication is characterized by interaction between sender and receiver. Two-way communication is used in most work situations. You should consider it your standard. Examples of two-way communication include

- casual conversations;
- arguments;
- on-the-job training;
- problem-solving meetings;
- counseling sessions;
- interviews;
- performance appraisals; and
- progressive discipline.

One-way communication goes from sender to receiver only—there is no opportunity for a response or a question from the receiver. One-way communication is used

- to give orders during emergency situations.
- in making an announcement over a public address system.
- with voice mail.
- when you send a memo.

The main disadvantage of one-way communication is that the sender can't check to see if the message was received as intended.

ACTIVITY

1. On a separate sheet of paper, list examples of one-way communication. Consider work, family, social, educational, and recreational situations.

2. On another sheet of paper, list examples of two-way communication. Consider work, family, social, educational, and recreational situations.

3. Place your two lists side by side. Note the characteristics that the items on the first list have in common with each other. Note the similarities among the items on the second list. Note how the two lists differ.

The examples you wrote for the first list (one-way communications) probably have at least one of two things in common: Either the information needed to be conveyed very quickly, or it was so routine in nature that no response was needed. In one-way communication, there is no way for the sender to make sure the message was received accurately. One-way communication is used most appropriately in situations where there are crucial issues to deal with such as in a cardiac emergency or when an information needs to reach as many people as possible in a short time.

The second list—two-way communications—probably contains examples of situations for which accuracy and common understanding are the primary needs. When senders and receivers need to solve a problem or reach agreement about an issue, two-way communication is the choice. Giving each other feedback about what was communicated allows people to compare what they intended to say with what was heard, to check their own understanding of what was said, and to correct any mistaken impressions (Bradley, 1990).

FACTORS AFFECTING COMMUNICATION

In any given communication, the receiver will probably understand somewhat less than 100 per cent of the facts, ideas, and feelings that the sender wants to communicate. A number of factors—the level of verbal and listening skills, the existence of physical barriers, our "perceptual filters"—can contribute to this deficit. Considering these factors can help make your communications clearer and more effective.

Verbal Skills

Sometimes it's not what you say, but how you say it that counts. Take the following sentence: "Will you get Mr. Conner's chart? I need to enter some notes concerning a conversation we had about his wound care after discharge."

The speaker can convey meaning beyond the meaning of the words with body language, emphasis, timing, facial expression, and pronunciation. The next activity will help you see how verbal techniques can change the meaning of the sentence above.

ACTIVITY

1. Ask another nurse or co-worker to help you with this activity. Without telling your helper what the "hidden meaning" or emotion is that you are attempting to portray, repeat the following sentence: *"Will you get Mr. Conner's chart? I need to enter some notes concerning a conversation we had about his wound care after discharge."*

Use different tones of voice to express

• contempt;

- anxiety;

- anger;

- excitement;

- cool detachment;

- self-confidence; and

- uncertainty.

Use the dictionary for clues if you're not sure of the exact meaning of a word or phrase. Add a word or two if necessary, but keep the sentence essentially the same. Have your helper evaluate how well you did by guessing the hidden emotion or meaning behind the words. Ask your helper to talk about the impact of receiving such a message from a nurse supervisor.

2. Add body language and facial expression when you repeat the sentence. Have your helper guess the hidden emotion or meaning behind the words. Notice whether your helper's accuracy improved or worsened.

Physical Barriers

It pays to be sensitive to your environment. Physical barriers to communication can include

noise. The noise level in a hallway for example, could make it hard for nurses to hear instructions concerning patient care. If stopping the noise is not possible, you may have to move to a quieter area for shift reporting.

distance. As distance between sender and receiver increases, it takes more effort to communicate.

lighting. Too much or too little light can interfere with message reception. People usually need to see body language and facial expression to get the entire message.

In large organizations, too many people may try to communicate at the same time. Under these conditions, receivers become overloaded and cannot give adequate attention to any one message. Misunderstandings and delays may result.

The complexity of an organization also creates problems with communications. In health care facilities there is little or no communication among many of the health care professionals representing the different departments and clinical subspecialties. Nurses primarily communicate with other nurses and physicians with other physicians. A high degree of specialization in personnel and departments in the health care facility tends to set up barriers to communication even when the facility's staff members are diligent in trying to keep communication open (Bradley, 1990).

Perceptual Filters

Your perceptual filter is the way you see the world. Among other things, it is made up of your

life experiences. How it was for you growing up, whether you had supportive parents, whether you spent a lot of time during your high school years at the library, involved in sports, or at the local mall.

feelings. Feelings about the people you work with, and your attitude toward life in general. Is life challenging and fun, or a nuisance? Many people have a predominant emotional "style," for example, cheerful, angry, anxious, loving, overwhelmed, or content.

fears. Some people fear illness or death more than financial instability; others are afraid of being left alone; still others fear other people.

stereotypes. We all have them, even if we'd rather be free of them. The following are some examples of stereotypes: "Supervisors have no sense of humor." "Computer programmers are nerds." "Doctors have overactive egos." "Nurses are bossy." "Old people have difficulty hearing."

prejudices. Like stereotypes, prejudices exist despite facts that might contradict them. However, whereas stereotypes can be positive, prejudices usually assume a negative bias.

Prejudices can range from "old people are feeble" to ugly, false assumptions based on race, religion, color, sex and other characteristics.

self-image. Your self-image has a profound effect on how you hear—sometimes whether you hear-what other people say to you. Your self-image consists of whether you see yourself competently fulfilling life's many roles—as a parent, for example, or a sibling, spouse, worker, community member, friend, boy/girlfriend or hobbyist.

Both the communication we send and the communications we receive can be distorted by these perceptual filters—ours and those of the people around us.

ACTIVITY

Take a few minutes with pencil and paper to write down the elements that have shaped your perceptual filters. Be honest—no one is going to see this piece of paper except you!

1. Many people remember their parents repeating a favorite motto, like "Some things are better left unsaid," or "Don't be afraid to toot your own horn." Others were given specific advice about life—"Never buy anything on credit," for example, or "Don't wear long hair after age 30." Describe some of your parents' advice or behavior that shapes your view of life today. (Your reaction against your parents' views can shape your life as much [or more than] your acceptance of them.) For instance, you may find that you are suspicious of new people in your life because your father told you that most people are out to steal from others. Or you may be drawn to people who work hard because your mother worked hard, enjoyed working, and told you that "hard workers make good friends."

2. Describe the one experience of your adult life that has most shaped your attitudes about life and people. Describe its effect on your behavior at work.

3. Everyone fears something. Write about your biggest fear in life. (Some possibilities: Death or illness, loss of independence in old age, financial disaster, being rejected by others, being alone.) Tell how this fear influences your working life, your choice of jobs, and the way you deal with your co-workers.

4. Identify the stereotypes you hold and how you came to be aware of them. For instance, one nurse was surprised when another nurse disclosed to her that she was a recovering alcoholic. She realized her stereotype of alcoholics—recovering or not—did not include her professionally successful and well-balanced friend.

5. People with low self-images are sometimes uncomfortable or embarrassed at compliments, or they stick with jobs they feel certain they can do. People with high self-images usually like to challenge themselves at work, and usually feel a warm flush of satisfaction when complimented. Describe how your self-image reveals itself to others.

Differences in perceptual filters are a major cause of communication problems. If the sender

---

Example

Anita Anderson, the nurse supervisor, asked Janet Banks to organize the unit's annual holiday party. Anita had become the supervisor of the unit two months ago. Janet had just transferred from another unit five months ago.

Janet's experience with hospital parties had been somewhat negative. On her previous unit, more than one party ended up with too many people drinking too much and getting noisy and disruptive. It nearly always created bad feelings that carried over into working relationships. In an effort to avoid the fiascos she'd seen in the past, Janet planned a very simple party—cake and punch after work on a Thursday afternoon, just before an important departmental staff meeting.

Anita had an entirely different experience with annual holiday parties. On her unit, parties usually involved a huge pot-luck lunch. Staff who hadn't had time recently to chat with friends in other work units "caught up" during the party. Photos of children were passed around, stories were told, staff who'd been promoted were congratulated, and news about those who had left the unit was passed on.

When Janet reported her plans to Anita, she was annoyed. After talking it over with a fellow supervisor, though, she realized that she had made assumptions about Janet's ideas without checking them out. She decided to talk with Janet about her experience with unit parties and ask if she were open to suggestions for a few changes to her plans.

Anita and Janet were operating under two different sets of expectations regarding parties—expectations born of their own experiences. Had they discussed their expectations, they might have avoided some confusion. Unfortunately, we are often unaware of our expectations until the receiver of the message makes a mistake.

---

and the receiver have had similar experiences with an object or event, their perceptions may be quite similar. If their experiences were not similar, their perceptions may not be similar.

Extremely good or bad experiences with individuals, facility departments, or events may influence how you perceive them today and therefore, how well you communicate with and about them.

Example

Daniel Donovan, a nurse supervisor with 15 years of VA hospital experience, handed a new ward clerk a stack of unit vacation request sheets.

"Will you please burn some copies of these?" he said. He didn't mention that "burn some copies" was navy slang for "make some photocopies."

An hour later, on his morning break, Daniel discovered the ward clerk in the parking lot, carefully dropping papers one by one into a flaming wastebasket. Thinking fast, he knocked over the wastebasket, stamped out the flames and saved most of the requests. But he never used VA slang again without making sure his listener knew what he was talking about.

Cultural Barriers

Sometimes the differences in experiences and learning we take from our home or work cultures can create communication gaps.

Racial and ethnic heritage, where we grew up, where we live now, and amount and quality of education determine cultural background. It is often a primary cause of differences in learning and experience. Therefore, be aware of how your own cultural background influences the way you communicate. And, remember that the cultural background of others can influence the way they communicate with you and receive your messages (Kozier, 1998). For example

- in many Asian cultures, it is considered disrespectful to make direct eye contact, especially with a boss.

- in Arabic cultures, flowery phrases and strong words don't always mean what they seem. However, repeating a phrase or sentence several times is an indication of sincerity.

- being singled out for a reward for work well done is considered insulting in some Native American cultures.

While it is important to consider the cultural background of the people you work with, it is equally important to remember not to stereotype them. There is a fine line between the two practices.

Each person's perceptual filter creates assumptions and expectations. When the assumptions and expectations of two people don't match, their communications can fall apart.

ACTIVITY

Read each of the statements in the columns below. The statements in column 1 represent the best qualities of a good nurse supervisor. In column 4, you'll find statements representing undesirable qualities. Columns 2 and 3 are somewhere in between. Place a check mark in each box that best represents your own qualities.

1	2	3	4
People trust me with personal information.	People can usually trust me.	People usually can't trust me.	People run the risk of becoming an "item" in the gossip mill if they share feelings or other personal information with me.
My behavior is consistent.	I'm usually consistent.	I'm usually inconsistent.	People are never sure what I plan to do next.
I exude energy and enthusiasm.	I'm usually enthusiastic.	I'm usually bored or disinterested.	I drain energy from others.
I have a reputation for knowing what I'm talking about.	I usually know what I'm talking about.	I sometimes act like I know what I'm talking about, even if I don't.	I am known as someone who makes up information rather than admit I don't know much about a particular subject.
People see me as competent in my work.	People usually see me as competent.	People usually see me as not competent.	People see me as someone who hides behind the competence of my staff.
People know me as someone who talks to others as equals.	I usually address others as equals.	I sometimes "talk down" to staff.	People see me "talking down" to staff.

Sometimes it's hard to see how we need to improve. Consider sitting down with a trusted friend or family member and going over these questions. If you keep an open mind, you may get some unexpected insight into how others see you.

GUIDELINES FOR EFFECTIVE COMMUNICATION

Communication begins with a sender. As sender, it is your responsibility to make it possible for communication to occur. The following guidelines will help you do that.

Establish Credibility

Long before you decide to communicate a message to a given staff member, you lay the ground work for that communication and all the others that follow. Being known as trustworthy, honest, pleasant, and fair is the best way to ensure clear communications with your staff.

Learn about the Receiver's Frame of Reference

Think about the people with whom you want to communicate—about their cultural backgrounds and motivations for working and their frames of reference. Try to imagine how their frames of reference are likely to influence how messages are received.

The better you know your staff, the more your communications with them can be "customized" to their frame of references—and the better your chances are of getting your message across.

Choose Appropriate Communication Methods

Based on your understanding of the receiver's frame of reference, choose the best verbal and non-verbal methods for communications. Because many nurses work solely in one specialized area of the facility, they may not be "up-to-date" with all the language used in the facility. For example

- if you are the supervisor in the operating room, you might want to avoid terminology that is "surgery specific" when communicating with staff on the psychiatric unit.

- if you were raised in a culture in which people stand close to each other, be sensitive to those who need more physical distance.

- if you are dealing with someone from a culture that values obedience, be sure to ask about personal priorities before requesting overtime. Make sure it is clear the person has a choice. Avoid this problem when possible by asking for volunteers for overtime.

Organize Your Message

Ask yourself, "What do I want to say?" Write it down if it helps. To get to the core of the idea, think of how you would say it if you had only three minutes to get the message across.

Deliver the Message in a Respectful but Assertive Way

Assertiveness is expressing oneself confidently while respecting the rights of others. Always treat others with respect. This means never talk down or suggest that the other person's intelligence, competence, commitment, or attitude is lacking even if you truly believe that is the case. Assertive nurse supervisors are able to present their feelings and values and stand up for themselves without demeaning the values and feelings of others.

Assertive communication means

- being able to communicate thoughts and feelings in a way that protects the rights of all.

- feeling comfortable and in control of negative feelings.

- having a positive attitude about communicating honestly.

- communicating competence and self-confidence.

Assertive communication techniques include

- starting statements with "I."

- expressing your own thoughts and feelings "I feel you are..."

- including positive and negative data in statements: "I like the way you organized the work area, but..."

- avoiding generalizations like "We all think..."

- providing oneself with time to respond appropriately when another person says something negative with a statement like: "I need to think about this" (Kozier, 1998).

Ask for Feedback

Feedback is one of the most effective tools for bridging gaps in our communications with others. Ask the receiver for feedback on what you have just said. One nurse supervisor says, "I'd like to be sure I've been clear about this assignment. Would you tell me what I told you, so I can be sure I've told you what I wanted to tell you." That way, she doesn't offend staff by suggesting that they didn't understand.

PART TWO—LISTENING SKILLS

Good listening, like good speaking, takes conscious attention and practice. Listening to feedback can be one of the more challenging forms of listening.

Asking for feedback is one thing. Taking it in is another thing entirely. Some of the pitfalls that can block your reception of feedback are:

- You are too busy sending messages to pay attention to receiving them.

- You are afraid of unfavorable reactions.

- You see feedback—no matter how respectfully phrased—as a threat to your authority or control.

If any of the above descriptions fit you, you're in good company—many people have similar reactions to feedback. It's possible to be a good listener most of the time and still have a strong reaction under certain circumstances. Some people are sensitive about some of their personal characteristics—a need for strict organization, for example, or their performance on a less-than-favorite task. Others overreact to feedback in discussions with people who "push their buttons."

Most people find that it doesn't help to tell themselves not to have these attitudes and fears. Instead, they learn to set aside their feelings while hearing feedback and use specific listening techniques. A description of some of these techniques follows.

POSITIVE LISTENING RESPONSES

Positive responses are accepting and understanding. They don't evaluate, they don't blame, and they don't judge. They say to the speaker, I value your input. I want to listen to you. I want to understand what you are saying and how you are feeling. Positive responses include the following.

Restatement. This response focuses on the content of the speaker's message. You restate in your own words what you heard the speaker say.

Example

Bob Stevenson, one of your staff members at Evansville Memorial, is trying to decide whether to continue to work for the hospital.

"I like the security, benefits, pay, and friendships I've developed," he says. "On the other hand, I might advance more quickly working for a smaller rural hospital. I might also get more personal recognition for my work."

If you want to *restate* what you heard him say, you might respond, "You seem to see two alternatives—stay with this hospital or leave. So you're weighing security, benefits, pay, and friendships against slow advancements and personal recognition."

Reflection. For this response, you go a step deeper and focus on the speaker's feelings. You might talk about how you feel listening to the speaker or how you think you would feel in the speaker's place.

Example

A reflective response to Bob's statements might be, "I think I understand how you feel. You're a little confused and not exactly sure what you want. I found myself in a similar situation when I was offered this job—I know what you're going through. I'm willing to give you any information I have that might help you come to a decision."

Question. This response can increase your store of knowledge about the speaker and help expand the speaker's perspective.

Example

Supportive questions to ask Bob would include the following

"What do you consider to be the most positive aspects of working for Evansville Memorial? The most negative?"

"What are your broad goals for your career? Where do you want to be five years from now?"

NEUTRAL LISTENING RESPONSES

When accompanied by nonverbal cues that you are listening (steady eye contact, nodding, leaning slightly toward the speaker, etc.), neutral listening responses can be powerful methods of communicating your concern and interest.

Silence. Silence can be most effective. Don't forget that your body language speaks even when your mouth doesn't.

Noncommittal acknowledgment. You don't have to agree with a person's perspective to acknowledge it. Brief expressions that communicate understanding, acceptance of the speaker's feelings, and empathy include the following.

- "Oh," or "Oh?"
- "I see."
- "Really."
- "Interesting."
- "Mm-hmmm."

Door openers. You can show your interest and involvement by inviting the speaker to expand or continue. For example

- "Tell me more about that."
- "Let's discuss that."
- "I'd like to hear your thoughts about..."
- "Sounds like you have strong feelings about…"
- "Would you like to talk about it?"

Observations. A sensitive observation of an individual's behavior can help both of you understand feelings that haven't yet been expressed verbally. For example

- "You look sad."
- "You seem anxious and upset."
- "I think you're concerned about the time."

NEGATIVE LISTENING RESPONSES

Negative responses are precisely the opposite of positive responses—they evaluate, judge, and blame. They "put down" the speaker or deny the importance of the speaker's feelings and concerns. They carry an unspoken message that says, *You and your needs are unimportant to me.* Negative responses to avoid include the following.

Joke

This response makes light of the speaker's concern. Often it reflects the listener's anxiousness or discomfort. Sometimes people will make a joke in an attempt to get the other person to "lighten up." However, making a joke of a serious situation tells the speaker, *You are not worthy enough for me to take seriously.*

Example

A negative, joking response to Bob's concerns might sound like this:

"I sure wish that was all I had to worry about. Maybe you should have a little chat with the Director of Nursing. She may be able to help you with that personal recognition problem of yours."

Attack

This is a criticism. It focuses on the person and says, *You are at fault and to blame for your problem.*

Example

"What do you want, anyway? Someone to pat you on the head every time you give good patient care? You have to learn, management doesn't have time to coddle nurses. Nurses who have their acts together know that job satisfaction has to come from knowing they are involved in meaningful work."

Denial

The listener tells the speaker not to worry, or not to feel the way the speaker feels. This response tells the speaker, *There is something wrong with you for feeling the way you do. I don't want to take the time to listen to you.*

Example

"I can't see where you have a problem. You want to hear about problems? Go talk with Tina Smith. She's got a kid on probation, her husband just left her, and she's up to her ears in debt. You should be happy your life is running smoothly."

Advice

Sometimes people want and need advice. Most of the time—especially when someone is discussing a problem in working relationships—advice just gets in the way. As a nurse supervisor (or, for that matter, a friend, spouse, parent, or sibling), you serve best when you serve as a sounding board, facilitator, and one who clarifies. Offering advice can say to the speaker, *"You can't solve this yourself. I don't have time to help you work through this and find your own solution. I know more about this than you do."*

Example

"You will never find a small rural hospital as good as Evansville Memorial. If I were you, I'd just stick around and watch the job board. Take it from me—I've been with Evansville Memorial for six years. You just need to start applying for different openings, and something better will eventually come up."

SUPPLEMENTAL ACTIVITY

1. Schedule about 30 minutes with a nurse supervisor—your own nurse supervisor or someone else. Ask the nurse supervisor to talk with you about incidents or developments at work that shaped his/her communications skills.

EXAM QUESTIONS

CHAPTER 3
Questions 17–29

17. Skillful communicators are

    a. people who decided to develop their skills.

    b. rarely found in management jobs.

    c. born, not made.

    d. always promoted to management positions.

18. Which of the following words or phrases is defined as "the transfer of information?"

    a. feedback

    b. perceptual filter

    c. communication

    d. environment

19. Which of the following words or phrases is defined as "the physical surroundings in which communication takes place?"

    a. environment

    b. feedback

    c. perceptual filter

    d. communication

20. Which of the following words or phrases is defined as "a response to a message?"

    a. communication

    b. perceptual filter

    c. feedback

    d. environment

21. Two-way communication is characterized by

    a. conflict.

    b. lack of response.

    c. interaction.

    d. authority.

22. Jill has a vague feeling she is not doing well on the job even though she was told in her review sessions that she has been performing very well. What is a possible nonverbal communication problem that is causing Jill's concern?

    a. Her nurse supervisor told her she did not have to work overtime.

    b. She does not have a close friendship with her supervisor.

    c. Her nurse supervisor never looks her in the eye during reviews.

    d. She has heard that some of her co-workers are faster at their jobs.

23. Factors that affect communication include

    a. verbal skills, physical barriers, and perceptual filters.

    b. language barriers, hearing filters, and speech.

    c. complexity of an organization, body language, and facial expression.

    d. cultural differences, perceptual filters, and body language.

24. The main disadvantage of one-way communication is

    a. it takes a long time to send and a long time to receive.

    b. it can be used only in emergencies and over public address systems.

    c. the sender can't check to see if the message was received as intended.

    d. it is inappropriate for all working situations.

25. Which of the following words or phrases is defined as "the way in which each of us distorts messages?"

    a. feedback

    b. communication

    c. perceptual filter

    d. environment

26. Differences in cultural backgrounds can lead to _____ when they're not taken into account.

    a. promotions

    b. poor planning

    c. misunderstandings

    d. procrastination

27. People who block their reception of feedback may be

    a. hard to understand when they speak.

    b. immature or not well-adjusted.

    c. afraid of unfavorable reactions.

    d. not using good speaking techniques.

28. If you wanted to verify the meaning of something someone just said to you, you could

    a. use feedback to paraphrase your understanding of what was said.

    b. analyze the meaning of what the person said.

    c. see if others around at the time heard the same thing you did.

    d. act on what you thought you heard and see what happens.

29. Another co-worker said to Joyce, this place really stinks, I think the management around here abuses the staff for kicks." Joyce responded with, "You seem upset; we should take a few minutes and talk." Which listening responses was Joyce delivering?

    a. restatement and feedback

    b. noncommittal acknowledgement and reflection

    c. observation and reflection

    d. noncommittal acknowledgement and door opener

CHAPTER 4

RELATIONS WITH NURSING STAFF

INTRODUCTION

Now that you know a little about some basic communication skills, you'll learn how those skills are applied. You'll learn how effective nurse supervisors give direction to their staff, how to plan a meeting and lead it, and how to keep your meeting moving.

CHAPTER OBJECTIVE

After studying this chapter, you will be able to recognize guidelines for directing staff and planning and conducting effective meetings.

LEARNING OBJECTIVE

Upon completion of this chapter, you will be able to:

1. Recognize effective feedback.

2. Identify the types of verbal direction.

3. Recognize the components of complete directions.

4. Identify the steps in planning a meeting.

5. Recognize the elements of conducting a meeting.

6. Recognize techniques for dealing with challenging meeting situations.

7. Recognize methods for encouraging participation in meetings.

8. Identify the maximum number of people that should attend a problem-solving session.

LESSON CONTENT

Communicating with your nursing staff requires not only an understanding of the theory of communications, but also knowledge of what types of situations occur when specific communication skills need to be applied. To be a skillful communicator—and thus a respected and skilled nurse supervisor—you must be able to apply good communications theory in real work situations.

GIVING FEEDBACK

In Chapter 3, you learned to ask for feedback. After you've communicated your message, asked for feedback, and listened carefully to what was said, the communication process reverses. Now it's your turn to give feedback.

Uses of Feedback

Feedback has three uses:

- **To verify the meaning of something said.** For example, you may say to someone who just gave you a piece of information, "Let me see if I understand the situation…," followed by your paraphrased version of what the person said to you.

- **To maintain behavior.** Giving feedback to staff whose performance has improved usually makes them aware of their effort.

- **To correct behavior.** You can give feedback to someone about their behavior when the behavior has been inappropriate in hopes that the person will change the behavior. For example, if you supervise Liz, who has been taking an extra 15–20 minutes at lunch break for the past week, you will want to provide her with feedback about how her tardiness burdens the nurse who is caring for her patient while she is at lunch.

Content of Effective Feedback

The content of effective feedback focuses on behavior. It is important to focus on what a person does rather than on our opinions of what that person is. Rather than calling someone a "loudmouth," you might say, "You talked more than anyone else in the meeting." Saying a staff member is "dominating" is probably not as helpful as saying something like, "Just now, you were looking out the window and yawning while others were talking. You didn't seem to be listening, but I felt I had to agree with your arguments or face attack from you." It is not appropriate to comment on a person's physical characteristics.

Shares information rather than advises. Sharing information leaves people free to make their own decisions in accordance with their own goals and needs. Information to share can include your understanding of other information, your positive or negative reactions, descriptions of praiseworthy or unacceptable behavior, and positive or negative consequences of behavior.

Considers the needs of the receiver. Feedback can be destructive when it serves our own needs for power or control or to "blow off steam." Define the purpose of the feedback before you give it. Feedback should be given to

help (either the work unit or the individual), not to hurt. Too often, people use feedback to "cut someone down to size." You can avoid this temptation by trying not to give feedback when you're really angry. Instead, take the time you need to calm down and work out your frustrations in whatever way works for you—exercise, talking it out with a friend, playing an instrument or working at a craft or hobby.

Doesn't overload the receiver. When you give more than the receiver can absorb, you are probably satisfying your own needs rather than helping the other person. One or two items of feedback at a time is usually enough.

Doesn't guess at other people's motives. Telling people what you think their motives are is usually guaranteed to create resentment. It is dangerous to assume you know why someone said or did something. "You just expect everything to go your way," is an invitation to a fight. However, if you are uncertain about why someone said or did something, your uncertainty itself is important feedback and should be revealed: "I can't figure out why you keep asking for things."

Characteristics of Effective Feedback Delivery

Once you've determined the purpose and the content of the feedback you want to deliver, you need to think about the delivery itself. Your feedback is most likely to be effective if it is

solicited. Feedback is most useful when the receiver actively seeks feedback.

well-timed. Immediate feedback is usually most helpful—depending, of course, upon the receiver's readiness to hear it, the support available from others, etc.

checked. One way to check your feedback for clear communication is to ask the receiver to rephrase the feedback. This way, you can see whether it corresponds to what you had in mind. No matter how good your intentions, feedback can be scary for many people. Because of that, people sometimes distort or misinterpret what others say.

GIVING DIRECTION

As a nurse supervisor, one of your main duties will be to accomplish quality patient care through others. This means you'll need to give staff direction and talk with them about what needs to be done.

Two Types of Direction

As with most skills, there is more than one way to give direction. In this course, we'll consider two ways to give direction to staff: You can tell them what to do, or you can ask them to do it.

Ask Them

Most nurse supervisors prefer working with this category of direction. There are two ways to ask staff to do something.

Request for input. Many nurse supervisors rely upon this method almost exclusively. When they have a problem or a job that needs to be done, they'll get their unit staff together, describe the situation and ask for solutions. They serve as meeting leaders, helping others participate in the decision-making process.

Appeal for volunteers. This is a good way to deal with extra assignments—overtime, messenger errands, serving on task forces, attending meetings as the unit representative, etc.

Tell Them

This type of direction has three subcategories.

Command. This type of direction is used sparingly—largely in emergencies or life-or-death situations.

Request. A veiled command. The request ("Would you do this?") doesn't leave the staff member with much more choice than

the command.

Suggestion. This allows for some difference of opinion from the staff member ("I'd like to see the shift report done this way. Do you think this method will be more efficient?"), but is still a "tell them" method of direction.

Anatomy of Direction

Regardless of the situation and the individual, good direction has a number of characteristics. A discussion of these characteristics follows.

The Four Ws. Every direction you give to a staff member should contain the answers to the following questions

- WHO?
- WHAT?
- WHEN?
- WHERE?

Sometimes direction also should include answers to the following questions

- HOW?
- WHY?

It's also a good idea to check for impact (did Brenda already promise to help someone else with a

---

Example

You are the charge nurse on second shift in an Intensive Care Unit where Brenda Wood is a staff nurse. It has been a frenzied afternoon, and the unit is in disarray. Brenda has a light assignment today, so you want her to coordinate end-of-shift straightening up of the unit. Your direction to her should include the following

WHO:	"Brenda, I need…"
WHAT:	"…someone to coordinate shift clean-up…"
WHEN:	"…by 2 p.m. today."
HOW:	"Ask each staff nurse to help you with the area around their patients' rooms."
WHY:	"It needs to be completed by 2 p.m. so that it does not interfere with end-of-shift charting."

lengthy procedure?) and for understanding (remember what you learned about seeking feedback).

ACTIVITY

Your hospital surgical unit has recently received supplies for the clean utility room. Enough supplies to fill the cabinets have been neatly stored away, the half empty boxes have been piled up around the utility room, getting in the way and presenting a fire and safety hazard. There is room to store them down the hall in storage room 52, which has been designated for overflow of supplies. The boxes are not heavy. You know that two staff nurses (Bob and Sharon) and the ward clerk (Linda) have the time to stack and carry the boxes to storage.

Write out the directions you would give to get this piece of work accomplished. Then check your answer against the one in the following box.

Feedback for Activity

If your answer resembled this sentence: "Would someone move the boxes piled up in the clean utility room?" your direction specified *WHAT* (move the boxes), but left out *WHO, WHEN, WHERE, HOW,* and *WHY.*

"Bob, I wish you would move the boxes piled up in the clean utility room to storage room 52" is a better answer. It specifies WHO, WHAT, and WHERE. It leaves out WHEN, HOW, and WHY. In some cases, these elements might not be important.

"Bob, the clean utility room is too cluttered. Would you move out some of the boxes that are piled up?" This direction contains WHY (clutter) and WHO (Bob), but omits WHAT, WHERE, WHEN, and HOW.

"Bob, do you have time to get help from Sharon and Linda and move the boxes piled up in the clean utility room to storage room 52 by noon?" This is probably the most complete direction you could give. It contains all the elements except WHY (which may not be important in this case): WHO (Bob, Sharon, and Linda), WHAT (move the boxes), WHEN (by noon), WHERE (to storage room 52), and HOW (with the help of Sharon and Linda).

General Rules

Besides the Four Ws, some general rules to keep in mind when giving direction include

- be sure the direction is necessary.
- be sure you have authority to give direction.
- be brief.
- be specific.
- request feedback and check for understanding.
- follow up.

PLANNING A MEETING

The effective nurse supervisor learns how to plan, conduct, and evaluate meetings and develop the art of constructive participation. You can make meetings work by planning each one according to these four steps (remember the acronym PAWS).

Step One: Define the Purpose.

Step Two: Develop the Agenda.

Step Three: Decide Who should attend.

Step Four: Select and schedule the meeting room.

Step One: **Define the Purpose**

If you know what you want to achieve during your meeting, it is likely to go quickly and to leave participants with a sense of accomplishment. To define the purpose of your meeting, determine whether you want to

- give or receive progress reports.
- conduct a training session.
- conduct a planning session.
- solve a problem.
- present new information to the group.
- listen to recommendations on a specific issue.
- discuss an issue.
- combine several functions.

Then ask yourself, "What would happen if I didn't call this meeting?" If the answer is "Nothing," or if your purpose could be better served with a memo, a one-to-one discussion, a telephone conversation, or some other method, then don't hold a meeting. If the result of not holding a meeting is less effective patient care, staff dissatisfaction, increased cost to the health care facility, or some other undesirable situation, then go ahead with your meeting plans.

Step Two: Develop the Agenda

This is your plan of action for the meeting. It summarizes the Five Ws—Who, What, When, Where, Why.

The agenda should note the meeting's purpose; the place, time, and date; when it should begin and end; and what presentations will be made and who will make them. Whenever feasible, distribute your agenda in advance. Meetings tend to go more smoothly when participants know what to expect and can bring relevant materials with them.

Step Three: Decide Who Should Attend

The meetings you conduct as a nurse supervisor will tend to have a "fixed membership:" you, the nursing staff, and ancillary help. However, when a problem arises that affects other units or departments, consider involving other people in your meeting. Even when a problem or decision has little effect outside the unit team members, you can occasionally get a different slant on issues by inviting a knowledgeable person from outside the group.

On the other hand, you may have to leave out people who expect to come to your meetings. Should this occur, use tact.

The success of a meeting depends not only on whether the right people attend, but on how many attend. A good rule of thumb is to invite no more than 15 people for a problem-solving session. If you must have a larger group, plan a lecture or a panel discussion. Large groups tend not to create the sense of individual responsibility that smaller groups do. Also, a large group doesn't allow full participation of each participant and can be a strain for meeting leaders.

Step Four: Select and Schedule the Meeting Room

Choose a room that's as comfortable and convenient as possible. If you plan to have a small meeting, don't hold it in a large room. On the other hand, try not to crowd people into small rooms. Make sure the seating is properly arranged and that equipment and materials necessary for conducting the meeting are ready.

CONDUCTING THE MEETING

Use the following five guidelines to generate effective and well-organized meetings:

- Start on time.
- Introduce the meeting topics.
- Follow the agenda.
- Stop on time.
- Follow up.

Start On Time!

When you start meetings on time, you send a clear message to everyone who is supposed to attend that they are expected to arrive on time. If you wait for stragglers, you reinforce the idea that your 2:00 meeting will start at "around two." Pretty soon, you find yourself starting close to 2:30. Avoid all that by starting on time, every time.

Introduce the Meeting Topic

Your opening remarks should focus the group's attention. Take no more than five minutes—more time increases the chances the group will begin to function as a passive audience rather than active participants. Begin the meeting by going over the agenda. Invite meeting participants to clarify any items they don't understand and to suggest additional agenda items. Explain that you want the group's ideas, but you won't put people on the spot by calling on them individually.

Follow the Agenda

Use the problem-solving model you learned in chapter 2 for any agenda item that requires a decision. Make sure the group understands each issue. Clarify and summarize when necessary. When the group gets off track, gently bring it back to the item under discussion.

The first response. The first response to an issue may be an important contribution, or it may be completely inappropriate. Your reaction to this first response can serve to encourage or discourage the group's further responses. Give no indication of approval or disapproval—just show you're glad that the person has spoken.

If appropriate to the purpose of the meeting, use a chalkboard, white board, or flip chart pad to record responses.

Follow-up questions. Don't take the first response as final, even if you are pleased with it. Use follow-up questions to keep the discussion going and encourage others to contribute. Follow-up questions can be simple:

- "What do the rest of you think?"

- "Does the group agree with this response?"

- "Can you elaborate on that, Chris?"

- "We've heard from the nursing staff. What do the ward clerks think?"

- "Has anyone besides Allison had experience with a case like this?"

- "Can you expand on that?"

Don't ask for ideas from people who haven't volunteered them. Don't go around the circle for responses. This practice frequently embarrasses those who cannot think of something to add to the discussion. Remember those who *did* offer ideas—when you refer to the ideas later, use the name of the person who made the suggestion.

Intermediate summaries. When you see an area of mutual agreement—that is, overlapping ideas where both sides partly agree—take advantage of them. Point them out. Sum up the area of agreement and ask for a consensus. Record the consensus.

Be careful, though—DO NOT TRY TO CONVERT THE MINORITY TO THE MAJORITY'S OPINION! You may not be able to get a unanimous vote—that's okay.

Further responses. As you receive more ideas, continue recording them. If you receive several different answers, pick the one that most closely fits the objective and develop it.

If the group tries to pass responsibility back to you by saying, "What do you think about this?" or "What is the correct answer?" pass it back to them with something like, "What is your idea on this?"

Conflict is okay. While discussions about matters that produce copious disagreement can cause discomfort, many times they yield wonderful ideas. Staff morale increases when plans are made to resolve any problem that causes a lot of discontent or stress.

As interest in the topic rises, however, control of the meeting can become more difficult. Because many staff members want to give their opinion, and some will bring up other topics of contention while they are speaking, discussions often get off the agenda topic. Here's where the good relationships you've built with your staff pay off. If the meeting participants respect you outside the conference room, they'll respect you inside, and give heed to your guidance.

Try some of these methods to get back on track:

- Stand up and be silent.

- Ask members to talk one at a time.

- Make a summary statement: "Let's review."

- Ask for help in getting back to the agenda item.

  Once you have a consensus, don't allow the group to keep discussing the issue. If you see that an item cannot be resolved because more facts are needed or an essential person is missing, don't waste time on it. Table the question for further discussion at a later meeting.

  At the end of each agenda item discussion, give—or ask someone else to give—a summary. Summaries bring a sense of closure and provide a chance to clear up any confusion.

Stop on time. Indicate to the group what has been accomplished. Close the meeting on a positive note. Review decisions and appoint committees for unsettled questions. Set a time for the next meeting, if appropriate.

Follow up. Your role as meeting leader doesn't end when the conference room empties. Good meeting leaders practice good follow-up principles to make sure the meeting's accomplishments aren't wasted effort.

If minutes were taken at the meeting, check them for accuracy. They don't need to be a transcript. The minutes summarize the following:

- Time, date, leader, or chair.

- Names of people attending.

- Agenda items discussed.

- Other items discussed.

- Decisions reached.

- Responsibilities assigned or taken.

- What time the meeting ended.

- Scheduled date, time, and place for next meeting.

Distribute copies to participants and other appropriate parties as soon as possible after the meeting. Others who should receive copies of minutes might include your manager, or nurse supervisor, people who were invited but unable to attend, and people whose work will be affected by discussions or actions in the meeting.

If you have agreed to initiate a change based on decisions made by the group, be sure you follow through. If others have agreed to initiate a change, meet with them to establish a timeline for carrying out their responsibilities.

LEADERSHIP CHALLENGES WITHIN MEETINGS

Thorough preparation and good meeting leadership skills don't always produce an effective meeting. Sometimes, meeting situations present challenges that stretch your diplomatic abilities. You can anticipate some of these challenges by studying the discussions on the following pages.

The Group

Each group, like each individual, has a personality. Being an effective meeting leader means determining the group's personality and responding appropriately.

Bright, active, responsive group. Think of this group as a spirited young horse. You don't want to break its spirit, but you have to control it enough to keep from being bucked off and trampled. You can accomplish wonderful results with this type of group—or be a flop. To make a success of a meeting with this group, be sure to

- be well prepared.

- give them questions fast.

- ask tough questions to slow them down.

- be firm.

- don't let them lead you.

- lead the group but encourage interaction.

Resistant, antagonistic group. Explore the cause of the resistance. Check for misconceptions and correct them if possible. Accept the group feelings and listen to their gripes, rather than resisting or arguing. Be empathetic to their concerns. Use any legitimate means to focus them on problem solving. Think of their resistance the way an eastern martial arts instructor might think of it: As a source of energy that can't be stopped by force, but can be harnessed and used by a skillful leader.

To harness the group energy you should:

- Face the situation frankly and ask why.

- Find one or two staff members who may be responsive and use them to help swing the group.

- Find an angle of the topic that may create personal interests.

- Use factual questions.

Slow, apathetic group. Their apathy may be due to inexperience, lack of understanding, or lack of interest. Thoroughly explain the topic. Again, use any legitimate means to get their interest. Think of the group as a sleeping giant; your job is to wake up the giant and get it moving. Some wake-up techniques include

- asking simple questions you know they can answer.

- feeding them information, then asking leading questions.

- displaying lots of energy.

- finding a common ground on which to meet them; building from there.

- asking thought-provoking questions.

- getting one or two talking.

- asking members what the resistance or hesitancy is about.

The Participants

While most staff members' participation in meetings is well-intentioned, it can sometimes pose a problem for the meeting leader. Staff members with strong personalities can derail a meeting if you're not prepared for their unique ways of contributing.

One universal technique is helpful with any staff member whose behavior is making problems for you: Speak to the person privately and explain how his or her behavior influenced the meeting.

Another way to deal with disruptive meeting participants is to practice "participatory leadership." This means concentrating on interactions with participants who respond, contribute, collaborate, and generally behave appropriately. By doing this, you create an atmosphere of constructive work and trust. Some suggestions for this interaction include

- link people's names with the ideas they offered.

- build on ideas offered.

- rotate the leadership of the meeting.

- delegate, empower, and encourage participation of meeting members.

- rotate recording duties.

- call on the specific skills of the participants.

Below are descriptions of eight common meeting personalities whose unchecked behavior can bring your meeting to a halt: Dominator, Helpful One, Sidetracker, Snoozer, Arguer, Dreamer, Chronic Critic, and Quiet One. After each description you'll find suggestions for tactful responses.

Dominator

Talks too much. Sometimes even takes control of the meeting away from the leader. Can take 20 minutes to say what others can say in one minute.

You don't want to stop this person from contributing; you just want to make sure everyone else gets a chance to talk, too.

Interrupt a Dominator's monologue with, "That's great. Let's get someone else's idea on that point," or "Your first point was that LVNs shouldn't be given post-surgical patients until the second postoperative day. Now, who else has an idea on this subject?"

- Give a Dominator a task: Recording secretary or listing ideas on the chalkboard, for example.

- Suggest politely that others may have something to say.

- Speak to Dominators in private; ask their help in drawing others out and suggest they speak less often.

Chatty One is a subcategory of the Dominator. This person carries on private conversations or argues points with the person in the next chair. To keep a Chatty One from destroying a meeting:

- Stop the proceedings, wait for the group to come to order. Establish eye contact with the Chatty One and smile.

- Say, "I am concerned that we are going to miss your ideas on this subject. Would you share them with us?"

- Say, "I'd like to hear from everyone, one person at a time."

Helpful One

Eager, bright, knows all the answers and wants to share them. May grow up to be a Dominator.

Some ways to deal with a Helpful One include

- smile, say thank you, and say you'd like to get other opinions.

- smile and ask the Helpful One not to make it too easy for the others.

- ask the Helpful One to summarize.

- make the Helpful One recording secretary.

Sidetracker

Diverts the group from the subject. Sidetrackers focus on their own agendas or go off on tangents.

You can help a Sidetracker stay on track by

- saying, "The meeting's straying off the agenda. Let's get back on the main issues."

- restating the problem under consideration.

- say, "This subject is interesting, but we'll have to take it up at another meeting. Let's include it on the next agenda."

Snoozer

Sleeps through the meeting. When awake, is bored. Does not contribute.

If it is a one-time problem, ignore it. However, chronic Snoozers should be talked to in private after the meeting—it could be physical. A chronic Snoozer who doesn't snore may just have to be ignored. For occasional Snoozers, try these methods.

- Call a break.

- Put the Snoozer on a committee.

- Consider not inviting Snoozers to your meetings.

Arguer

Likes to argue for the sake of arguing. Arguers believe they are helping others see both sides, but usually they just bring everything to a halt. Share characteristics with the Dominator.

You can blunt the Arguer's effect on the group with these techniques.

- Ask the Arguer if you can proceed to the next issue since this one seems to be at a standstill.

- Ask Arguers for their help.

Dreamer

Has a favorite theory. Likes to expound on them. If no favorite theories, has a habit of making totally impractical suggestions.

To bring a Dreamer back down to earth

- ask for substantiation of a favorite theory.

- analyze one of the theories-with a smile.

- call on the Arguer.

- ask the Dreamer to develop, write up, and present a favorite theory, perhaps for a Suggestion Award.

Chronic Critic

Sees no purpose in meeting. May be angry. May not be feeling well. May be unhappy in their jobs.

- Be especially gentle with these staff members.

- Encourage the Chronic Critic to make a constructive contribution.

- Meet privately with the Chronic Critic to uncover the issue.

Quiet One

May appear bored. May be shy, afraid of ridicule, hesitant to say something the boss may hear about later. Would rather just listen. May lack self-confidence; may be a Chronic Critic in disguise. Quiet Ones could be members of cultures that frown on speaking up in public.

To draw out the Quiet One

- play up to the Quiet One's interests.

- call on the Quiet One's experience with a topic under discussion.

- while looking directly at the Quiet One, ask the group a question you know the Quiet One can answer.

- when you do get a response from the Quiet One, give him or her a verbal pat on the back.

- use a direct question as a last resort.

- protect the Quiet One from any hint of ridicule.

- give Quiet Ones tasks you know they can accomplish.

You

After a meeting, evaluate your performance as a leader. Use the list from the following Supplemental Activity to help you.

SUPPLEMENTAL ACTIVITY

After conducting a meeting, use this form to evaluate your performance.

EVALUATION OF MEETING OF _____(Date)

1. Objectives met at this meeting: _____

    _____

2. Objectives not met at this meeting:_____

    _____

    Reasons they weren't met: _____

    _____

3. What I did especially well at this meeting:____

    _____

    _____

4. Aspects of my meeting leadership that need work: _____

    _____

    My plan for working on these aspects (for example, attending a seminar on meeting skills, practicing with family or friends before the next meeting, making notes on 3″ × 5″ cards, starting earlier on meeting plans, etc.): _____

    _____

    _____

    _____

5. Things I will do differently during the next meeting: _____

    _____

EXAM QUESTIONS

CHAPTER 4
Questions 30–43

Questions 30–31 refer to the situation described in the paragraph below.

Maureen wanted a unit secretary, Jaime, to find some medical records. She said to him, "Jaime, I need the last admission chart for a client named Mr. Andrew Glen, Client I.D. number 354-78-9982. Would you request the chart from medical records and put it on my desk?"

30. What element was missing from Maureen's direction to Jaime?

    a. when

    b. what

    c. who

    d. where

31. What is the best way for Maureen to make sure that Jaime understands exactly what she wants?

    a. "Jaime, do you understand what I said? You know that sometimes you don't understand."

    b. "Please repeat to me what I just said to you so that I know that you know what I want."

    c. "Now, would you tell me what I told you? I want to be sure I didn't leave anything out."

    d. If Maureen stated the direction clearly, she shouldn't need Jaime to reassure her that he understood.

32. Feedback is most effective when it is

    a. quick, to the point, and loud enough to be heard clearly.

    b. solicited, well-timed, and checked for clear communication.

    c. creative, given quickly, and provides advice.

    d. thorough, done at a leisurely pace, and kindly spoken.

33. There are two types of direction. They are

    a. "Tell Them" and "Ask Them."

    b. "Command" and "Request."

    c. "Suggestion" and "Appeal for Volunteers."

    d. "Order" and "Request."

34. Many nurse supervisors rely exclusively on one method of giving direction. That method is

    a. command.

    b. request for input.

    c. appeal for volunteers.

    d. suggestion.

35. What information does the acronym PAWS give about meetings?

    a. how to plan them

    b. when to have them

    c. how to behave at them

    d. how to avoid them

36. Which of the following is the first step in planning a meeting?

    a. select and schedule the meeting room

    b. decide who should attend

    c. define the purpose

    d. develop the agenda

37. Which of the following is the third step in planning a meeting?

    a. select and schedule the meeting room

    b. define the purpose

    c. develop the agenda

    d. decide who should attend

38. A good rule of thumb for a problem-solving session is to invite no more than _____ people.

    a. 10

    b. 15

    c. 25

    d. 30

39. What are two of the five basic elements that allow you to conduct a meeting smoothly?

    a. Allow a "brainstorm of ideas" session and stop on time.

    b. Do not stick too closely to the agenda and allow 5-minute breaks.

    c. Allow everyone to speak and keep the meeting short.

    d. Start on time and follow the agenda.

40. The important thing about the first response to the topic at a meeting is

    a. it is usually totally inappropriate.

    b. your reaction to it can encourage other responses.

    c. it should not be taken too seriously.

    d. you should write it down immediately on the board.

41. To encourage participation during a meeting, you can

    a. keep the agenda short.

    b. provide minutes from the previous meeting.

    c. use questions and summaries.

    d. allow the group members to talk for as long as they wish.

42. If you're leading a meeting that gets off the agenda, you can help bring it back by

    a. using the gavel.

    b. leaving the room for a few minutes.

    c. talking louder than anyone else.

    d. making a summary statement.

43. Jerry holds a weekly unit meeting. One of the staff nurses, Becky, nearly always sleeps through each meeting. Which of the following is the best way for Jerry to handle this situation?

    a. Report the problem to the Unit Coordinator and document your meeting results.

    b. Interview other nurses on the unit to see if they know why Becky is having difficulty staying awake.

    c. Write a memo for the entire staff about staying alert during unit meetings and detail the disciplinary actions you will use to correct the problem in the future.

    d. Speak with Becky about her problem, then refer her to the Employee Assistance Program if necessary.

CHAPTER 5

BUILDING COOPERATION WITH NURSING STAFF

INTRODUCTION

Learning how to build a team requires a basic understanding of cooperation. This chapter begins by explaining the meaning of cooperation and its importance in accomplishing nursing unit goals. After a discussion of two types of individual cooperation—vertical and horizontal—the chapter moves on to group cooperation and ends by comparing groups and teams.

CHAPTER OBJECTIVE

After studying this chapter, you will be able to identify ways to build cooperation and teamwork among nursing staff.

LEARNING OBJECTIVES

Upon completion of this chapter, you will be able to:

1. Recognize the importance of cooperation/teamwork.

2. Recognize the definitions of horizontal and vertical cooperation.

3. Identify appropriate ways to cooperate vertically and horizontally.

4. Identify the benefits of group membership.

5. Differentiate between groups and teams.

6. Identify ways to create a team from a group of individuals.

7. Recognize signs of poor cooperation in a nursing unit.

LESSON CONTENT

In any health care facility, quality patient care is accomplished only through the efforts of many people. All health care facilities need staff who can cooperate and nurse supervisors who can secure the willing cooperation of those working for them. The ability to cooperate with and get cooperation from others is extremely important in supervision (Tappen, 1995). Successful nurse supervisors understand and practice the principles discussed in this chapter.

WHAT DOES IT MEAN TO COOPERATE?

Walk into a health care facility and you can almost "feel" whether the spirit of cooperation is present or not. You can see it in the faces of the people, in the appearance of the workspace, in the reception you receive, and in the way the work is performed. Poor cooperation is indicated whenever bickering, jealousy, and friction are present. Absenteeism, frequent accidents, indifference, sloppy work, griping, criticism of management, "buck-passing," loafing, high turnover, poor planning, lack of or indifference to training—all of these are danger signals indicating lack of cooperation.

Cooperation means working together with another individual or other individuals to achieve a common goal. Cooperation is based on good human relations and on an understanding of human behavior. Individuals able to cooperate with one another usually have

- an ability to share responsibility and credit with others.

- flexibility to accept, overlook, or adapt to individual differences.

- an ability to listen to the contributions of others and see the relevant points.

- an ability to provide and receive feedback constructively.

Cooperation is the responsibility of everyone on the job. Nurses and other health care facility staff cooperate with co-workers and with their supervisors. Nurse supervisors cooperate with upper management, other nurse supervisors, and with their staff. All staff members cooperate both vertically and horizontally.

VERTICAL COOPERATION

Vertical (up-and-down) cooperation refers to your relationships with upper management and with those you supervise.

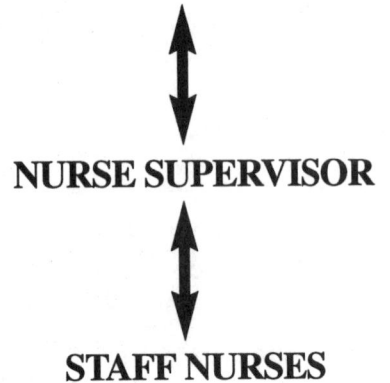

UPPER MANAGEMENT

NURSE SUPERVISOR

STAFF NURSES

Successful nurse supervisors satisfy their bosses and, at the same time, motivate their staff so that they will maintain high-quality patient care. They are concerned with relationships in both directions.

Cooperating with Your Boss

To build and maintain a cooperative relationship with your boss, you need to pay attention to a few basic concepts:

Commit yourself to the nursing department and unit goals. Make yourself as knowledgeable as possible about the goals set for the nursing department and your unit. Keep up to date on any changes. It is up to you to help your staff understand these goals and work toward accomplishing them.

Keep your boss informed. Share good news with your boss. It is important for your boss to know when unit operations are running smoothly and when your people are performing well. You and your unit's staff deserve the recognition, and it will help maintain your boss's perspective when things aren't going too well.

Share the bad news with your boss too. This doesn't mean sharing every gripe or problem that comes up. It does mean letting your boss know when you foresee major problems. Don't wait until the problem is out of hand! Also, honestly admit any misjudgments you may have made. It is better for your boss to find out from you than from others. Accepting responsibility for your own actions conveys a much better impression than finding excuses or blaming someone else.

Support your boss. Many experienced nurse supervisors rate loyalty as number one on the list of desired qualities. The loyal staff member is an individual worthy of trust and one who supports management in word and in practice. As a loyal nurse supervisor, you should

- PLACE YOUR BOSS IN THE BEST

POSSIBLE LIGHT WITH OTHERS! Don't criticize your boss in front of your staff, your peers, or other personnel. You will not only lose the trust of your boss, you will lose the trust of those around you.

- Support your boss's decisions. You may express your disagreement with your boss in a respectful way, but once a decision is made, you need to drop the issue and support your boss's decision.

- Maintain a positive attitude. If you allow a negative attitude to show through, you will infect those around you. Your staff members look to you for cues as to how they should think and act.

Keeping these basic concepts in mind, evaluate the behavior of the nurse supervisors in the activity box below.

ACTIVITY

Ronda Jones and Trang Nguyen are both nurse supervisors. They have been called in by their boss, Irma Lopez, to work together on a project. They both disagree with the way Irma wants them to implement the project, but neither says anything during the meeting.

After the meeting, Ronda goes back to her unit and complains to her staff about how the boss is out of touch with the "real world." When Trang goes back to his unit, he sits down and organizes his thoughts. He looks at why he disagrees with Irma and comes up with a couple of alternatives he thinks are workable. He then sets up an appointment with Irma so that he can discuss his ideas with her.

Decide which of these nurse supervisors you would want working for you. On a separate piece of paper, write a paragraph explaining why.

If you are like most people, you picked Trang over Ronda. By criticizing her boss in front of her staff, Ronda could damage her reputation in Irma's eyes and in the eyes of her employees. If Irma hears about Ronda's remarks, Ronda may find it very difficult to gain Irma's confidence in the future. It may also undermine the trust Ronda's staff has in her. Even if they agree with her assessment of Irma, they cannot help but wonder if Ronda criticizes them behind their backs too.

Trang's behavior, on the other hand, is very constructive. He avoids criticizing Irma in front of others. Since he has some positive alternatives to suggest, he also avoids sounding like a complainer when he talks to his boss. If Trang's ideas are well-thought-out, Irma may go along with one of them.

Cooperating with Staff

Maintaining a cooperative relationship with staff is as important as maintaining a cooperative relationship with your boss. To win the cooperation of staff, you need to apply many of the same principles you apply in maintaining a good relationship with your boss. Staff need to be able to count on you to stand up for them, keep them informed, provide suggestions and feedback tactfully, and set a positive example for them to follow.

HORIZONTAL COOPERATION

Horizontal cooperation refers to your relationships with your peers—fellow nurse supervisors, nursing staff, and other personnel.

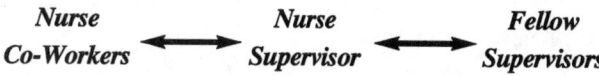

| Nurse Co-Workers | ⟷ | Nurse Supervisor | ⟷ | Fellow Supervisors |

As a nurse supervisor, you will need to build cooperative relationships with other nurse supervisors. Although you may find yourself in competition with some of these people for recognition and for higher positions, it will be to your benefit to cultivate an atmosphere of cooperation. When choices for key jobs are made, the individual who is able to foster and maintain harmony in all of his or her relationships *will* be given highest consideration.

Working cooperatively with other nurse supervisors requires attention to a few simple rules:

Demonstrate a willingness to cooperate.

Voluntarily supply experience and knowledge other nurse supervisors can use. Share information and ideas whenever it is appropriate. Remember, feedback is most effective when it is solicited.

Look at the example that follows. It is the same example as was shown earlier, with one important difference.

ACTIVITY

Ronda Jones and Trang Nguyen are both nurse supervisors. They have been called in by their boss, Irma Lopez, to work together on a project. They both disagree with the way Irma wants them to implement the project, but neither says anything during the meeting.

After the meeting, Ronda goes back to her unit and complains to her staff about how the boss is out of touch with the "real world." When Trang goes back to his unit, he sits down and organizes his thoughts. He looks at why he disagrees with Irma and comes up with a couple of alternatives he thinks are workable.

When he sets up an appointment with Irma, he suggests that they include Ronda in their discussion, since she too will be involved in carrying out the project. Irma agrees.

On a separate sheet of paper, describe what Trang did differently this time.

This time Trang took the initiative to include Ronda in the second meeting with Irma. By doing so, he demonstrates his concern for maintaining good relations with Ronda. He knows that he would not like to be left out of a planning meeting.

Respect the Other Nurse Supervisor's Territory.
Close working relationships with other nurse supervisors can be a challenge, particularly when there is an overlapping of functions. Cooperating in this type of situation requires respect for the "territorial rights" of the other individual. To enhance coordination and minimize friction, sit down with the other nurse supervisors and

- decide what tasks and responsibilities involve both supervisors.

- decide the priority of the tasks.

- coordinate task assignments.

- set up clear lines of authority.

It is essential to set up ground rules with the other nurse supervisor(s) before assigning tasks to staff. If it is not clear what tasks must be accomplished, which tasks must be done first, who is responsible for accomplishing the tasks, and who the staff members report to, chances are there will be confusion and friction among staff and nurse supervisors and the job will not get done.

Keep criticisms of others to yourself. Every time you are inclined to criticize a fellow nurse supervisor, particularly in talking to your nursing staff, restrain yourself. If you demonstrate respect for others, your staff will have a greater respect for you, for the organization as a whole, and will be inclined to follow your example.

Accept responsibility for your own actions.
Accepting responsibility is as important in horizontal relationships as it is in vertical relationships. One way to acquire a poor reputation among your peers is to always blame someone

else for everything that goes wrong. People will have more respect for you if you explore ways to correct mistakes instead of blaming others. After all, the important thing is to minimize the damage and ensure that the same mistake doesn't happen again.

ACTIVITY

Beth Peterson has been a supervisor (clinical coordinator) on the OB-GYN ward for one month. During this time, she has developed a good relationship with the nursing staff. They appreciate the fact that she hasn't rushed in to change everything. They also like the fact that she is easy to approach with their concerns. However, during this month, Beth has been so busy getting used to the job and getting to know the nursing staff, she hasn't seen much of her boss and hasn't had a chance to get to know any of the other clinical coordinators.

Check the type(s) of relationships Beth needs to spend more time developing.

___Vertical

___Horizontal

If you checked both vertical and horizontal, you're right! Remember, vertical relationships refer to up and down cooperation. Beth has developed a good relationship with her staff, but not with her supervisor. And, she hasn't focused any attention on her horizontal relationships with other clinical coordinators.

Maintaining strong vertical relationships with upper management, your immediate boss, and your staff and strong horizontal relationships with your peers and fellow nurse supervisors is essential to your success as a supervisor. Take every opportunity—chance contacts, performance reviews, staff meetings, phone conversations, and so on—to build and reinforce good human relations both inside and outside your department.

GROUP COOPERATION

Now that you are familiar with the importance of individual cooperation in the workplace, let's look at groups and how cooperation can turn groups of individuals into productive teams.

Benefits of Groups

Primitive people initially banded together in groups to protect themselves from the dangers of a primitive world. Alone, individuals were vulnerable and nearly defenseless. Together, individuals gained strength and could exert power against hostile forces.

People soon discovered that safety was not the only advantage of banding together. There were other physical benefits, such as

- shared resources and skills.

- ability to govern and influence others.

- participation in group recreational and ceremonial functions.

There were also psychological benefits, such as

- feelings of security and a sense of belonging.

- a collective identity and sense of purpose.

- pride and a feeling of accomplishment.

Many groups exist in today's world that satisfy the same needs and provide the same types of benefits. There are political, religious, and professional organizations; and there are recreational clubs, cliques, and gangs. Think for a moment about your work environment and about the community in which you live. Then complete the activity that follows.

ACTIVITY

Think about the kinds of groups you, your nursing co-workers, and members of your family belong? On a separate piece of paper, list as many of these groups as you can.

What Is the Difference Between a Group and a Team?

Group behavior and cohesiveness vary depending upon the purpose of the group, the type of leadership the group has, and the reasons individuals join the group. Some groups are loose, and the members have very little personal interaction. Exercise clubs are a good example of "loose groups." Other groups are so tightly knit that the members do not feel secure and cannot make decisions without one another. Gangs are good examples of these kinds of **groups.**

Groups that exist to achieve a specific goal or a series of objectives require more from their leaders and participants. Organizations that need to accomplish business, community, and governmental functions are good examples of these kinds of groups. Organizations such as hospitals and health care clinics require leaders who elicit cooperation and commitment from their staff members. They also require staff members willing to work cooperatively in a problem-solving process. In other words, health care facilities require groups that work as **teams.**

Looking at the table that follows, compare the characteristics of teams with the characteristics of groups.

As you can see, cooperation is the cornerstone of teamwork. In a team, members recognize that personal and team goals are best accomplished through cooperation and mutual support. When a team leader fosters a secure environment, members feel comfortable in expressing ideas and opinions openly. Members contribute to goal accomplishment by combining their unique knowledge and skills with those of other group members. They feel pride in the final decisions that the team leader makes because those decisions are based on their ideas and suggestions.

GROUP MEMBERS	TEAM MEMBERS
• Are passive participants	• Are active participants
• Work independently	• Work together
• Focus on themselves	• Focus on a common goal
• Leave responsibility for reaching goals to others	• Take responsibility for accomplishing the team goal
GROUP LEADERS	**TEAM LEADERS**
• Encourage conformity	• Encourage individual ideas and contributions
• Control the flow of information	• Encourage open exchange of information among team members
• Encourage passive participation of members	• Encourage active participation of members
• Foster a climate of competitiveness	• Foster a climate of trust and openness

ACTIVITY

Look at the groups you listed. Place a T next to the ones that are teams. For each one that is a team, list the characteristics that make them teams.

Building a Team from a Group of Individuals

One of your primary jobs as a nurse supervisor is to guide the efforts of those working for you toward accomplishing unit and nursing department goals and objectives. How successful you are in this endeavor will depend on how successful you are in building a team from a group of nurses with different backgrounds, motivations, values, and goals.

SUPPLEMENTAL ACTIVITIES

1. a. List the people in your department/unit with whom you have or should have a vertical relationship.

    b. List the people in your department/unit with whom you have or should have a horizontal relationship.

2. Look around you at work. Observe your behavior and the behavior of your co-workers.

    a. Make a list titled "Cooperative Behaviors." Under this title, list all of the behaviors you have observed that demonstrate a willingness to cooperate.

    b. Make another list titled "Uncooperative Behaviors." Under this title, list all the behaviors that indicate an unwillingness to cooperate.

    c. On the second list, note the behaviors that you yourself display. Of these behaviors, check the ones you think you can change into cooperative behaviors.

CHAPTER 5
Questions 44–51

44. Excessive absenteeism, accidents, loafing, indifference to training all indicate

    a. poor cooperation within the unit.

    b. an active, vital workplace.

    c. lack of health care facility regulations.

    d. an understaffed unit.

Question 45 refers to the conduct of Jane Sutter described in the paragraph below.

Jane was promoted to clinical coordinator of her unit a couple of months ago. Since then, she has developed good relationships with the staff nurses of the unit. They are happy with her unhurried approach to changes in the unit and with her openness about their concerns. She has met with her new boss once during the past two months and hopes to find time to get together with other clinical coordinators sometime next month—after she feels more settled in her new position.

45. Which statement applies to Jane's activities at work?

    a. Jane needs to spend time developing both vertical and horizontal relationships.

    b. Jane needs to spend time developing vertical relationships.

    c. Jane needs to spend time developing horizontal relationships.

    d. Jane is doing an adequate job of developing both vertical and horizontal relationships.

46. What type of cooperation refers to your relationships with your peers?

    a. group cooperation

    b. vertical cooperation

    c. horizontal cooperation

    d. staff cooperation

47. Donna says, "It makes me feel safe and secure, like there's somewhere I'll always belong. It gives me a sense of who I am and what I'm doing here in this life. Also, I'm proud of its work in the community." What is Donna talking about?

    a. her new job as a nurse supervisor

    b. the benefits of belonging to a group

    c. the stress-reduction technique she practices with others

    d. the advantages of working for the health care facility

Question 48 addresses the situation described in the paragraph below.

Diane was appointed to direct a project team of seven staff nurses. None of the people on the team know each other. Diane chats with each of the team members individually and notes that Karla, another staff nurse, seems quite shy. At the first team meeting, Diane introduces each of the team members and points out their qualifications. When Karla makes a suggestion for changing shift report procedures, Diane writes it on the board and asks Karla for more details.

48. What team-building principles is Diane using?

    a. She is establishing a chain of command, with herself at the top.

    b. None so far; she needs to examine her methods and start organizing.

    c. She is encouraging open communication and individual participation.

    d. She is leaving the responsibility of reaching goals to management.

49. Nurses in supervisory positions should

    a. argue with their bosses to show them the other side of issues.

    b. never disagree with their bosses in public or private.

    c. support their boss's decisions.

    d. be a sounding board for staff nurses.

50. Team leaders, unlike group leaders, tend to

    a. encourage conformity.

    b. foster a climate of competitiveness.

    c. encourage active participation of members.

    d. leave responsibility for reaching goals to others.

51. Team members, unlike group members, tend to

    a. focus on themselves.

    b. be passive participants.

    c. control the flow of information.

    d. work together.

CHAPTER 6

RELATIONS WITH CLIENTS

INTRODUCTION

In the past decade, health care reform has brought about cost cutting measures which have been frequently challenged and criticized by the public, politicians, and industry leaders. Today, health care facilities are very concerned about the sometimes negative views people have about health care organizations. Many clients and their families come to the health care setting with anxiety concerning the quality of care and treatment they will receive. You, as a nurse will need to be especially sensitive to their concerns and you will need to use your best communication skills with both families and clients.

Although clients are our first concern, the communication skills used in dealing with our clients are also used in dealing with clients' families and the public. For brevity's sake, we will use the term client to represent clients and clients' families and the public (our potential clients).

Applying communication skills in dealing with the clients you serve is not much different from applying them to dealing with nursing staff. The main difference is the amount of time available for making an impression. You have 40 hours a week to build relationships with your staff, while a five-minute conversation may shape a client's opinion of the health care facility staff, and the health care facility as a whole, for years to come.

In this chapter, you'll see how you can ensure that your unit's nursing staff members are making the best impression. You'll look at the benefits of good client relations and the nurse supervisor's role in maintaining them. You'll also learn some practical tips for making a lasting good impression.

CHAPTER OBJECTIVE

After studying this chapter, you will be able to recognize ways to improve and maintain good client relations.

LEARNING OBJECTIVES

Upon completion of this chapter, you will be able to:

1. Identify barriers to communication between clients and nurses.

2. Recognize the benefits of good relations with clients.

3. Identify the role of the nurse supervisor in maintaining good client relations.

LESSON CONTENT

The staff members of most health care facilities are made aware of their personal responsibility for promoting good client relations. Here's how courteous and helpful service benefits your health care facility.

- Good client relations create community support for health care facility growth.

- A good reputation attracts talented nurses, physicians, and administrators.

- Good client relations attract more clients to the health care facility.

WHAT ARE "CLIENT RELATIONS?"

Client relations includes everything the health care facility does that has an affect on clients' attitudes and actions, including:

- Health care services provided to clients.

- Direct care rendered to clients.

- Health care facility programs provided to clients.

- Appearance of the health care facility, grounds, and equipment.

- Appearance, attitude, and actions of health facility staff, *on or off the job.*

The Nurse Supervisor's Role in Client Relations

As a nurse supervisor, you may have more or less contact with clients than before you were promoted. Whether your client contact increases or decreases, however, you have new functions as a nurse supervisor. Nurse supervisors

- provide an example of good client relations whenever they do have contact with the clients.

- encourage and train staff who have client contact to practice good client relations.

Be aware of the unit's day-to-day activities and how they promote the health care facility's image. For example, each of the following affects how clients think of the health care facility:

- The quality of care the client received.

- How the unit's staff treats visitors.

- How the unit's telephone receptionist treats angry family members.

- The appearance of the unit.

- The appearance of the unit's staff.

ACTIVITY

On a separate sheet of paper, list the ways your unit's activities present a picture of the health care facility to clients. Review the list above for ideas.

OFF-THE-JOB CLIENT CONTACTS

Nurse supervisors are not responsible for the behavior of staff members outside working hours. However, supervisors can help make staff aware of how their behavior—on or off the job—influences client opinion about the health care facility.

ON-THE-JOB CLIENT COMMUNICATION

The physical setting of the health care facility and the organization of activities often hamper communication in the health care facility setting. Health care facilities are bureaucracies, and rules and policies common to bureaucracies tend to foster rigidity and create communication barriers.

There is also a tendency in health care facilities to place a higher value on the psychomotor aspects of nursing rather than the cognitive and feeling aspects of nursing. Therefore, nurses who are task oriented are rewarded over nurses who are people oriented. Other barriers to communication between clients and nurses include

- the use of technical language.

- rigid routines adhered to in health care facilities.

- a busy atmosphere.

- the clients' roommates.

- uniforms worn by staff.

- fragmented nursing care that clients sometimes receive.

- high noise levels.

As a nurse supervisor you need to set an example for your staff nurses and teach them to lessen the negative impact of these barriers to communication. The negative impact of the health care facility bureaucracy can be lessened by teaching your staff to:

- Use language clients can understand, and guard against health care facility jargon.

- Show genuine interest in clients by listening attentively, and remain aware of your nonverbal behavior. Diffuse the "I'm too busy to talk," message sent out by the busy facility atmosphere by sitting down beside the client and showing him or her you are ready to take time to listen.

- Allow clients as much choice as possible in order to make them feel more control over their daily care and activities. This includes increased flexibility with visitors when it is in the client's best interest.

- When the unit is noisy, keep the doors to rooms closed. Close the curtains around the client's bed before you talk with them so that your conversation can be private. Get close enough to sit by the client and speak quietly. Remember, the client may not talk freely if they feel the conversation is privy to every person in the room.

- Diminish the negative affects of the nursing uniform by treating the clients as active participants in their own care. Use problem solving, and encourage client feedback in your approach to client care.

TELEPHONE COURTESY

Staff members who answer a telephone on the job should learn rules for telephone courtesy. Nurse supervisors must check to be sure their staff members use the following guidelines in answering the telephone.

Answer with your unit name and your name (and your title, if appropriate).

- "Intensive Care Unit, Ms. Stevens speaking."

- Listen carefully to the incoming conversation.

- Answer questions carefully and clearly.

- Use a tone of voice that indicates a pleasant and eager-to-help attitude.

- Keep paper and pencil handy so that you can write messages or take down phone numbers without putting a caller on hold to search for supplies.

- If you need to put a caller on hold for more than 30 seconds to look up a document or answer a question, offer to call back in 10 minutes. Remember to do it. DO NOT put a caller on hold so that you can finish a conversation with someone else.

- If the caller asks for someone who is not in, check to see if you can help the caller yourself or take a message. Use a courteous phrase like, "Mr. Garner is unavailable. May I help you?" or "Mr. Garner is unavailable. May I take a message?"

- If you will be absent from your unit and someone else will pick up your calls while you're gone, leave a note by the telephone like, "To Trach Care Update Class. Sandra Corwin RN is caring for my patients in my absence. Back at 10 a.m. L. Garner RN."

- Keep voice mail announcements up-to-date and businesslike (Finch, 1995).

BILINGUAL COMMUNICATIONS

Englishis a second language for many residents in this country. Nursing staff should make sure language isn't a barrier to taking care of clients. Staff should be aware of people in their health care facilities who speak Spanish, Tagalog, Chinese, Vietnamese and other languages common to our culturally diverse country. In case they forget, remind them that speaking English LOUDER to someone who has difficulty with English won't help their understanding. Patience, and sometimes, repetition, are helpful. Be sure to speak slowly and use short sentences.

SUPPLEMENTAL ACTIVITIES

1. On a separate sheet of paper, make a list of all the people in your health care facility who are fluent in another language, as well as the languages they speak.

2. Next time you walk into your unit, walk in thinking, "What would I think of this health care facility if I were a client being brought by wheelchair into this unit for the first time?" Try to be objective. Write down all your negative and positive impressions. As a supervisor, what can you do to reduce the negative impressions?

3. Another day, walk into your unit and put yourself in the place of a client who is frightened about their diagnosis and really needs to talk. Be aware of the barriers to communication that you would perceive if you were this client. Write them down. Now think about solutions to these barriers.

EXAM QUESTIONS

CHAPTER 6
Questions 52–54

52. Community support and involvement, talented staff nurses, and public support for health care facility projects are all benefits of

    a. employment within the health care system.

    b. being a successful nurse supervisor.

    c. belonging to volunteer organizations.

    d. good relations and communications with the public.

53. The supervisor's role in maintaining good public relations is to

    a. report all examples of bad public relations to departmental head.

    b. be a good example and provide training and encouragement for staff nurses.

    c. hold weekly meetings on good public relations practices.

    d. write press releases about interesting developments in the unit.

Question 54 addresses the situation described in the paragraph below.

Mr. Reese is a 75-year-old male who was recently hospitalized for the first time. He was told to save his urine for 24 hours for testing. Mr. Reese told the nurse who explained the procedure that he needed help to stand to urinate. The nurse agreed to send someone in to help Mr. Reese to the bathroom and made a note on the client record. The nurse told Mr. Reese, "Use the call light when you need to void." Early that afternoon Mr. Reese called his wife and said, "I want to go home! I've been very patient but not one person has been in here to help me. That nurse said someone would be in here to help me go to the bathroom, and I've been waiting two hours to go!"

54. What is the problem in the situation described in the previous paragraph?

    a. Technical language caused a barrier to communication.

    b. Lack of detailed client teaching concerning 24-hour urine collection.

    c. The nurse was poorly trained on how to collect a 24-hour urine specimen.

    d. The patient had unrealistic expectations of the nursing staff.

CHAPTER 7

ORGANIZING AND PLANNING SKILLS FOR NURSE SUPERVISORS

INTRODUCTION

As a nurse supervisor, understanding the organizational structure of the rules, relationships, and lines of communication in your particular health care facility is imperative to your success. Additionally, understanding the organizational process or philosophy that your health care facility uses to provide patient care allows you to successfully plan and organize the overall nursing care of the patients/clients in your unit. However, since these organizational structures and patient care delivery systems are specific to each health care facility, we will not endeavor to cover them in this course. We will, however, cite generic organizational and planning skills a nurse supervisor can use in any health care facility environment.

This chapter is divided into two parts.

Part One: Organizational Skills

Part Two: Planning Skills

After your promotion to nurse supervisor, you will have more tasks to organize than ever before. Your job no longer consists of getting several tasks done in the space of a day. Now you'll have to make sure everyone else gets their tasks done in the allotted time. You'll need to know who is doing what, and when. This added responsibility calls for taking a step back and getting a wider view of your nursing unit goals than you had before.

Nurse supervisors have access to far more resources and will be responsible for far bigger projects than staff nurses. To keep track of all that information, you'll need a system. In this chapter you'll start out learning how to keep track of the people and other resources available to you. You'll learn how to set up three different kinds of filing systems and what kinds of documentation you'll need to keep on your own activities.

After learning the basics of getting organized, you'll learn how to create a daily and weekly job plan. You'll learn how to chart a plan for a new assignment or project, and you'll learn the importance of committees in the development and implementation of your plans.

CHAPTER OBJECTIVE

After studying this chapter, you will be able to identify ways to organize and plan activities in your nursing unit.

LEARNING OBJECTIVES

Upon completion of this section, you will be able to:

1. Recognize methods used to organize the activities of a unit.

2. Specify the four options you have for dealing with each document that comes to you.

3. Identify the elements of a daily job plan.

4. Identify the elements of a job plan for a new assignment.

5. Specify advantages and disadvantages of task forces and other committees and the informal organization.

PART ONE—ORGANIZA-TIONAL SKILLS

Nurse supervisors organize their own work, and they organize the work of others and coordinate that work with other individuals, groups, and resources. Without the foundation of good organizational skills, work efforts can collapse into chaos; with it, work can flow smoothly.

KNOW YOUR RESOURCES

Organized people who set out to complete a task always check their resources before beginning. You will have human resources from the medical, nursing, and allied health departments in the health care facility; and physical and technical resources from the building, the grounds, and the supplies and equipment available to you. All these resources will help you as nursing supervisors realize the goal of the delivery of quality client care.

These human and physical resources, however, can present an "information overload" for the nurse supervisor. How can you be sure you are using all the resources that will result in the highest possible client care, when just keeping track of your resources can be so overwhelming? The answer is, organizing the information you have into easily accessible and condensed documents that can be used as supervisors' job aids. Creating resource charts and flow charts is one way of developing this type of resource documentation. Today, many nurse supervisors use computers to assist them in the development of resource charts and documents. There are many software products available to help you. There are also hand-held computerized note-taking tools and computerized organizers. These may be used to help you keep your documentation and schedule current.

Employee Charts

Your most important resources are your human resources—the staff members who make up your unit and other people available to you from the nursing department and other departments in the health care facility. A staff chart will help you see at a glance who is in your unit, what each person's role, duties, and authority limits are, and how each person's position relates to the positions of the others in the unit. Following you'll see a sample staff chart. The chart shows the people available to supervisor Smith in the ICU on the day shift.

Sample Design for a Staffing Chart

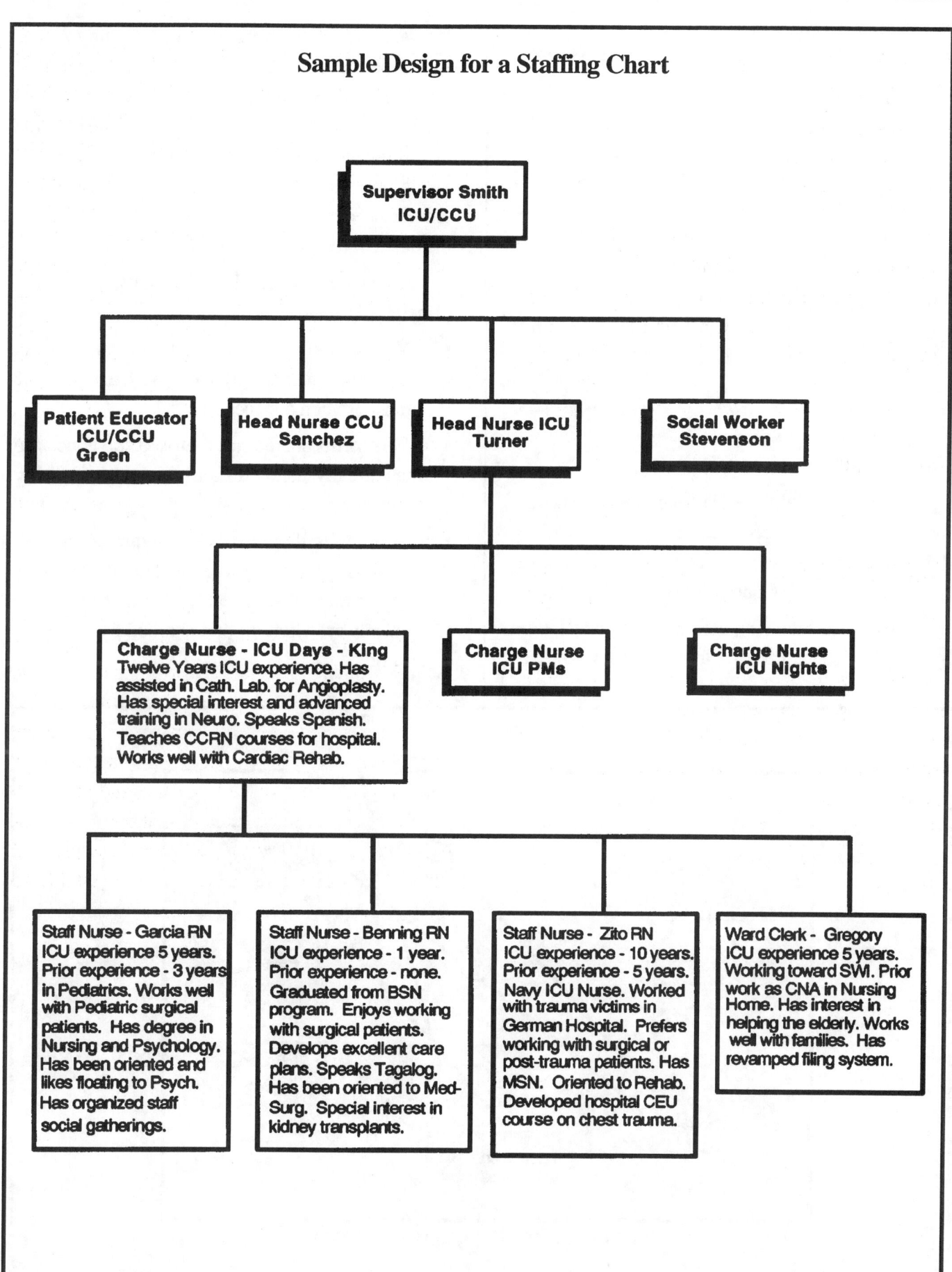

Supervisor Smith ICU/CCU

Patient Educator ICU/CCU Green

Head Nurse CCU Sanchez

Head Nurse ICU Turner

Social Worker Stevenson

Charge Nurse - ICU Days - King Twelve Years ICU experience. Has assisted in Cath. Lab. for Angioplasty. Has special interest and advanced training in Neuro. Speaks Spanish. Teaches CCRN courses for hospital. Works well with Cardiac Rehab.

Charge Nurse ICU PMs

Charge Nurse ICU Nights

Staff Nurse - Garcia RN ICU experience 5 years. Prior experience - 3 years in Pediatrics. Works well with Pediatric surgical patients. Has degree in Nursing and Psychology. Has been oriented and likes floating to Psych. Has organized staff social gatherings.

Staff Nurse - Benning RN ICU experience - 1 year. Prior experience - none. Graduated from BSN program. Enjoys working with surgical patients. Develops excellent care plans. Speaks Tagalog. Has been oriented to Med-Surg. Special interest in kidney transplants.

Staff Nurse - Zito RN ICU experience - 10 years. Prior experience - 5 years. Navy ICU Nurse. Worked with trauma victims in German Hospital. Prefers working with surgical or post-trauma patients. Has MSN. Oriented to Rehab. Developed hospital CEU course on chest trauma.

Ward Clerk - Gregory ICU experience 5 years. Working toward SW. Prior work as CNA in Nursing Home. Has interest in helping the elderly. Works well with families. Has revamped filing system.

ACTIVITY

Make your own staff chart. First check with the personnel department for job descriptions of each staff member in your unit, including yourself and your supervisor. Reduce each job description to a few words. Write each description and any other information you find helpful on a small, sticky-backed piece of paper. Arrange the pieces of paper on a large piece of paper, moving them around until you have them in the proper hierarchy for your unit.

Flow Charts

Often it is helpful to chart the physical movements of forms, material, or personnel. Anything that moves in a regular routine through a unit can be studied this way (Fisher, 1996).

Look at the following example of an ineffective motion flow chart. It shows the path followed by a laboratory technician who must make hourly rounds in an open four-bed burn unit. The technician must (1) pick up lab work requests at the ward clerks desk, (2) pick up any specimens obtained by the nurses that go with the requests, (3) have the supervising nurse record the time on the slip and verify that the specimen has been picked up and, (4) leave the unit to return the specimen to the laboratory.

In analyzing work flow diagrams, keep these principles in mind:

• Work should progress directly from unit to unit (or person to person) with the least possible transportation distance.

• Work items should not return to someone who has already handled them (except for quality control).

• Work items should move in sequence through the unit without zigzagging. This is especially important in an open bed unit where the patients are likely to be disturbed by increased traffic.

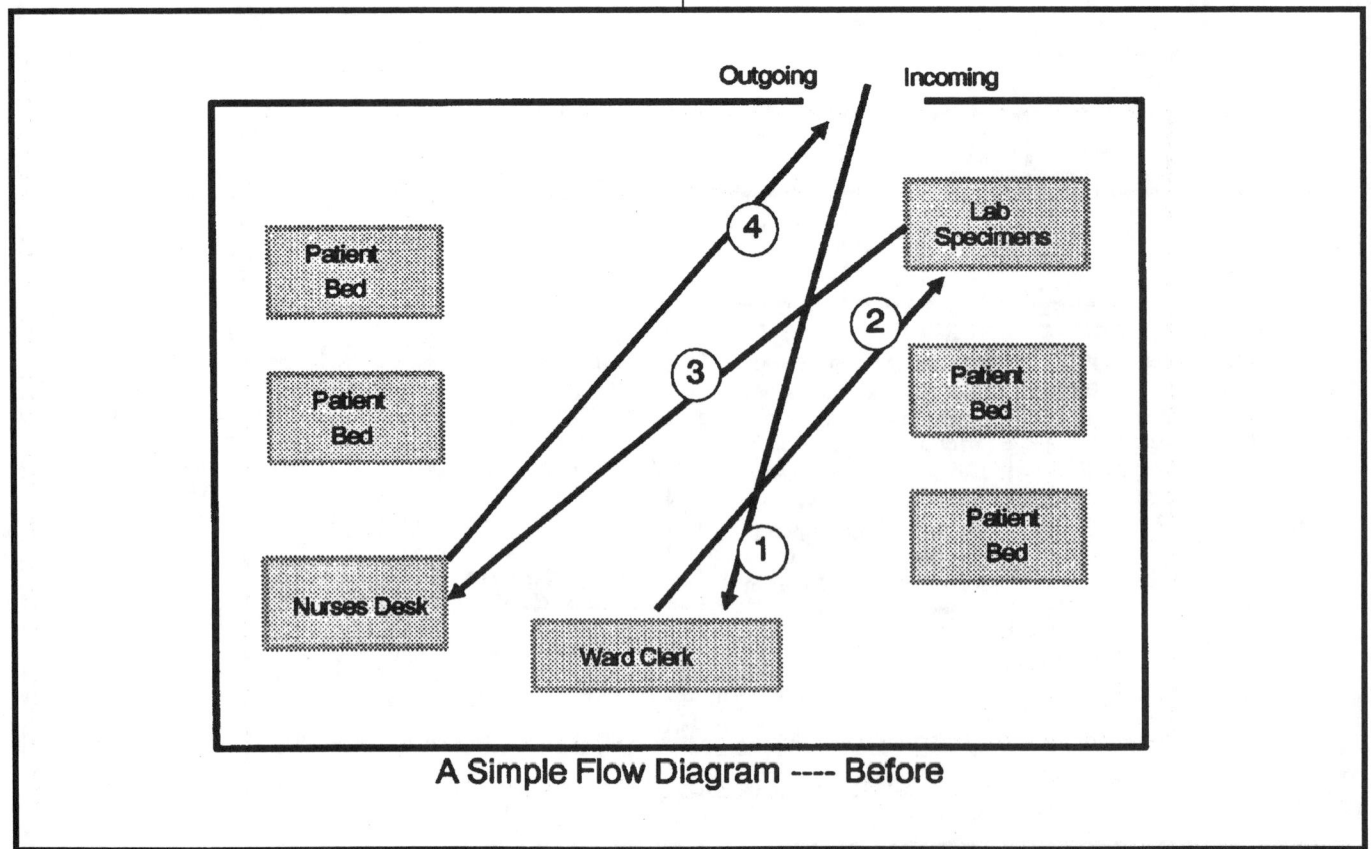

A Simple Flow Diagram ---- Before

When the diagram is analyzed, the weaknesses of the system become apparent. The laboratory technician has to cross the room to pick up requests prior to picking up the lab specimens that went with the requests. For quality control, the supervising nurse has to check when specimens leave the unit, and the technician has to cross the room again. Look at the diagram after the room has been rearranged to control traffic.

The changes needed to streamline the operation were simple. The desks and beds were rearranged so that no one has to cross the room to pick up a document or specimen. Placing the ward clerk's desk close to the door also has other benefits. Both visitors and other health care facility staff can check with the ward clerk about a patient's availability without walking to the far side of the room and creating the possibility of disturbing all the patients. The work flow for many health care facility staff from other departments becomes a simple matter of IN and OUT.

ACTIVITY

Choose one activity that takes place in your unit-the processing of a single document or form, or the performance of one task that is done by either staff in the unit or external health care facility staff. Create a flow diagram for the activity. List the ways the work flow could be improved.

FILES

Every nurse supervisor has paperwork. Efficient nurse supervisors use one or more of the following systems to stay organized. Your choice will depend on personal preference and the type of work you do.

No matter what filing system you use, you should go through it from time to time to weed out "deadwood" which are old files not of use to you

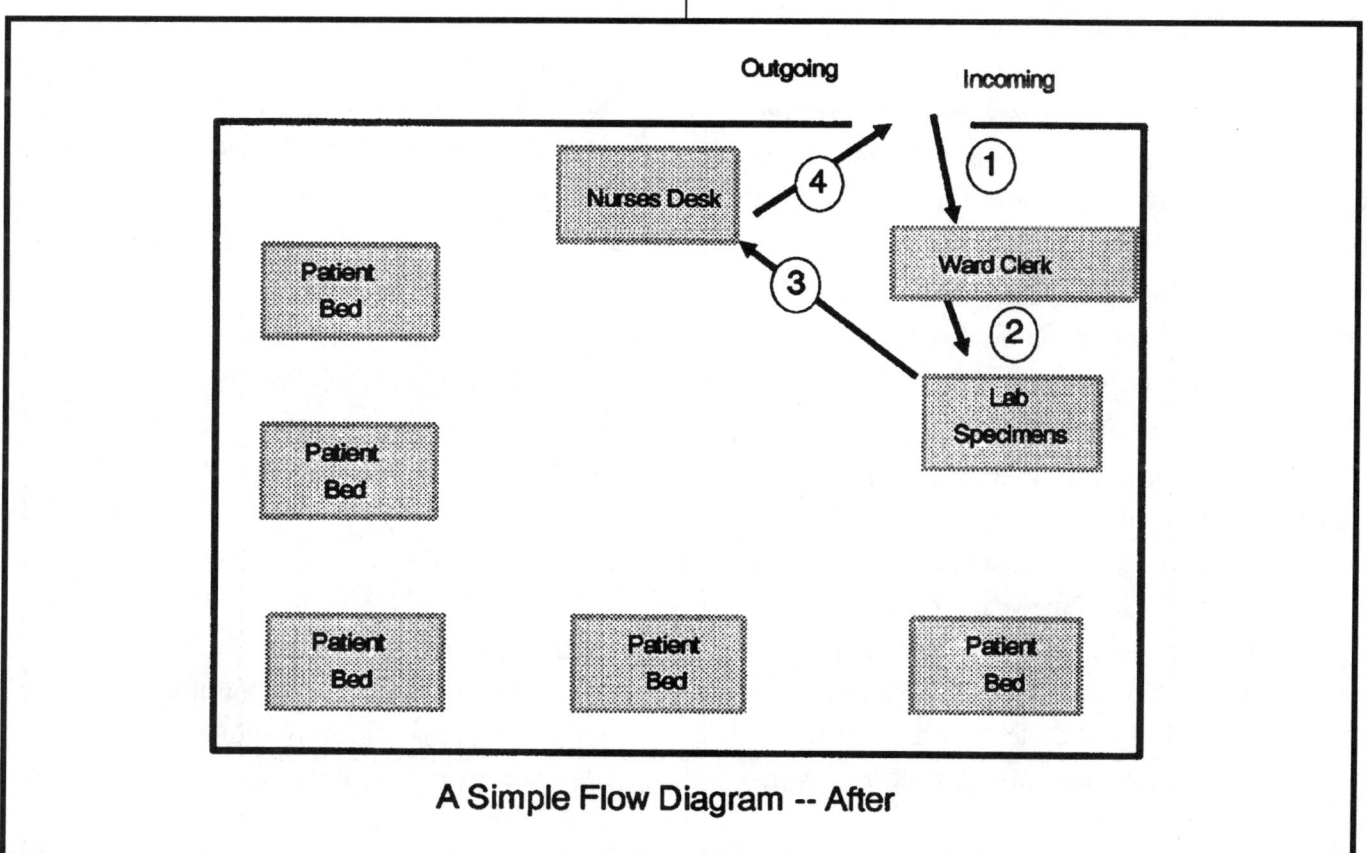

A Simple Flow Diagram -- After

anymore. You'll have less deadwood to deal with if you don't keep every document that crosses your desk or comes to you by e-mail. For each e-mail, memo, letter, clipping, or flyer that you receive, your four options spell FAST.

- File it for future reference.
- Act on it now.
- Send it on to someone else.
- Throw it away.

Tickler Files

Tickler file systems are designed to "tickle" your memory so you won't forget commitments and tasks that must be done on a particular date (Tappen, 1995).

The simplest tickler is a desk or pocket calendar or computerized organizer —many people prefer the kind with one day per page or screen. Use it to document every commitment you make. When you tell someone you will do something by a particular date, when you promise to call someone back, when you make an appointment or get notice of a meeting, write it down for the appropriate date. Also, write yourself a reminder several days before an important deadline. That way, you won't be surprised when you turn the calendar page one morning and see "Budget projections for next year due today."

When you meet a commitment, keep an appointment, or finish a job on deadline, check it off. Items remaining at the end of the day should be copied over onto another page.

A more elaborate tickler file is the 12-31 System. Label 31 folders "1" through "31" (for the days of the month) and a second set "1" through "12" (for the months of the year). Items that need to be accomplished on a particular date or within a particular month are filed in the appropriate folder. The key to making this system work is checking the appropriate folder each day and at the beginning of each month.

If you work on a computer, check with other experienced users to see what kinds of ticklers your software provides.

Alphabetical Files

You will receive notices, memos, requests, and other miscellaneous papers. For papers which you have no computerized files you will need to use paper filing systems. One practice followed by nurse supervisors is to keep these copies in an alphabetical file. Twenty-six file folders, labeled with letters of the alphabet and placed in a desk drawer nearby will help you find papers when you need them. For example, a notice on "Medical Leave" could be filed under "L" for Leave.

Personal Files

This is your own system, set up according to your needs and your own logic. Use a limited number of categories, and try to avoid the "Miscellaneous" designation—those folders somehow end up being the fattest ones. The following categories are useful starting points for many nurse supervisors:

Background Information. Separate folders within this category can be organized by topic. Refer to them when you need statistics, examples, or quotes.

Ideas. One or more folders can contain items to investigate that might improve your unit.

Miscellaneous Tasks. Miscellaneous tasks are small chores to be accomplished when you have a few spare minutes. Some people call this their "rainy day" file. Examples of miscellaneous tasks include cleaning up old computer files, weeding out old brochures and letters, and cleaning out your "miscellaneous" file.

Projects. Each folder corresponds to a project you are working on. Depending on the size of the project, you may wish to make each project a separate category, with file folders labeled according to topics.

Self-Development. This category has folders for items related to education and training, especially as it relates to your nursing interests.

DOCUMENTATION

As a nurse supervisor, you may sometimes be called upon to produce proof of a conversation or an activity. You may want to jog your own memory, or you may be asked to testify at a hearing. The best way to ensure that you can supply accurate information is to **Write It Down.**

This means documenting what you do each day. Keep a record that shows who you talk to, what is discussed, what tasks are accomplished, which tasks are assigned or delegated, what memos are written, what calls are received. It's usually not possible to record every single event. Get in the habit of documenting exceptions like exceptionally poor performance or exceptionally outstanding performance. Documentation is especially important in personnel matters, but remember that there may be disclosure requirements on personnel notes. Check with the nursing department personnel officer.

Notes don't have to be extensive or time-consuming. A word or two for each entry is usually all that is needed. In fact, some people who keep extensive notes in their calendars or "to-do" lists just save those. In many cases, these documents create a detailed diary.

For other, more complex contacts (such as performance appraisals), be sure to follow your department's recommended documentation procedures.

PART TWO—PLANNING

Planning is a future-oriented process that involves a whole set of interrelated actions applied for solving a current or anticipated problem. Proactive planning is done in anticipation of future or potential problems. Reactive planning is done in response to an existing problem.

Exxon manager Douglas Gehrman cited reasons for planning. These reasons include the following:

- Increases the chances of success by focusing on results, not activities.
- Forces analytical thinking and evaluation of alternatives, thus improving decisions.
- Orients people to action instead of reaction.
- Increases staff involvement and improves communications.
- Helps one discover the need for change.
- Is cost-effective.

DAILY AND WEEKLY PLANNING

Short-term projects or objectives can be best accomplished with daily or weekly planning. What goes into the making of a plan? For non-supervisory staff, it is sometimes fairly simple: you just write down what you plan to do today, or this week, and schedule your time accordingly. For nurse supervisors, it can be a bit more involved than that. It starts with research.

Check Your Resources

People preparing to accomplish a task must first check their resources-supplies, equipment, assistance available. Nurse supervisors preparing a plan must do the same things. Check the following resources:

Human Resources. Note who has what kinds of skills.

Equipment. Check to see that all necessary equipment is on hand, including safety equipment. Check to see that equipment is operational.

Supplies. Check to see that all necessary supplies are on hand.

If you find you are missing an important resource, take steps to replace it. This may mean submitting a requisition through proper channels, arranging for training or temporary help, or consulting with your supervisor.

Set Weekly and Daily Goals

It is human nature for people to want to be able to point to their accomplishments at the end of a day. For some tasks, it's easy to create daily goals. Others must be broken up into smaller segments to provide a measure of accomplishment.

Many nurse supervisors draw lessons from their experience in other jobs. They search their memories for experiences and use them to formulate plans to improve working conditions at their current health care facilities.

Weekly Goals

To set daily goals, it is necessary first to plan weekly goals. The form following this "Weekly Goals" section is designed to help you organize goals for you and your work unit and incorporate items from your tickler file. Follow the steps below to see how it is used.

STEP 1 At the top of the form, write the date the week starts.

STEP 2 Under that, write the objectives your unit is to meet during the week. Go back to your tickler file for objectives. For instance, this nurse supervisor's objectives are to collect time cards, conduct a unit meeting, complete next month's staffing schedule, and reorganize the clean utility room.

STEP 3 In the spaces below your list of objectives, write each task necessary to accomplish the week's objectives.

STEP 4 Rank each task according to its priority. Assign an A to tasks that must be done-those that are critical to completing your week's objectives.

Assign a B to tasks that should be done. These tasks are worth spending some time on—important, but not as critical as the A tasks.

Assign a C to tasks that could be done. These are tasks that are worth considering, but should be done only after the A and B tasks are completed. In some jobs, you may never get to the C tasks. Some people place their C tasks on a "Blue Moon List" or "Wish List."

STEP 5 Estimate the time it will take to accomplish the task, and note it in the appropriate space.

STEP 6 Assign a day for the task to be accomplished. Remember to assign tasks to days in the order in which they'll be accomplished. For instance, the work schedule can't be completed until after the deadline for all vacation requests has passed.

STEP 7 Using your staff charts, assign individual tasks to employees qualified to carry them out.

IMPORTANT

One role of the nurse supervisor is to help staff grow professionally. Use your knowledge of your staff's abilities and individual goals for growth to choose assignments that will help them stretch and reach their goals. Try not to get into the habit of giving the "best" assignments only to the "best" workers.

PLAN FOR WEEK OF _____

This Week's Objectives:

1. _____

2. _____

3. _____

4. _____

5. _____

Task	Priority (ABC)	Time to Complete	Day	Staff

Daily Goals

When your weekly plan is done, you're ready to begin on a daily plan. Some health care facilities provide forms to help you keep track of your daily plans. Also, daily goals may be noted on your personal organizer. Following this "Daily Goals" section are two examples of worksheets. No matter which form you use, it is important to:

- **Always check off tasks as you complete them.** Some people draw a line through completed tasks. Others place a check or X before the ones they've finished. Use whatever method makes you feel most satisfied, but don't skip this step. Not only do checks help you keep track of your progress, they give you a sense of achievement.

- **Keep your daily plan out where you can see it.** Your plan will do you the most good if it is posted where you can refer to it often or in your pocket organizer. Plans are only useful if they're consulted, and they're only consulted if they are easy to see.

- **Be sure to assign a priority to each task.** That way, when emergencies occur and you must sacrifice some tasks, you can quickly decide which ones to put off until later.

- **Follow up at the end of the day.** Tasks not completed during the day should be carried over to the next day, whether they were your tasks or tasks assigned to other staff members. Keeping track of your scheduling this way will mean you'll learn about your work habits and the capacities of the nursing staff. Your planning will become more accurate as you learn more. Some people find the end of the day to be a good time to plan for the following day; others prefer to make their daily plans in the morning.

- **Involve your staff in your plans.** Don't make your plans in isolation. One way to involve them is to meet with your staff on a regular basis to go over the work ahead, client care impact, methods of doing certain tasks, etc. You need their input, and they need to feel included. You will usually find staff more willing to cooperate with you when you consult them about planning decisions.

THINGS TO DO TODAY

Date:_____

Tasks to Complete	Done?	Appointments	
		8	
		9	
Phone Calls to Make	**Done?**	10	
		11	
		12	
People to See	**Done?**	1	
		2	
		3	
		4	

MONDAY			
Task		Appointments	Notes
		7	
		8	
		9	
		10	
		11	
		12	
		1	
		2	
		3	
		4	

CREATING A JOB PLAN FOR A NEW ASSIGNMENT

When you are given a major job or project that is new or unfamiliar to you, your planning becomes more complex. Begin by researching the project. Investigate the following:

- Purpose of the mission or plan.

- Equipment and supplies needed.

- Procedures and processes to be used.

- Staff needed for the project.

- Manuals and other publications related to the project.

- Special safety considerations.

- Extra training needed.

- Availability of current, qualified staff in your unit.

- Project deadlines.

- Need for coordination or cooperation with other units or departments.

If you write out all procedures and processes to be used in the project—safety procedures, paperwork processing, etc.—you're more likely to notice if something is missing or if a step has been skipped.

When your investigation is complete, you are ready to chart the project. The Action Planning Worksheet is designed for this purpose and is described below.

An action planning worksheet can be as simple as a list of steps required to complete a project. More complex worksheets include beginning dates, projected completion dates, cost estimates, and names of staff responsible for specific tasks. You can use this worksheet or design your own. In any case, refer to your research list (above) to fill it out.

ACTION PLANNING WORKSHEET

Objective: _____

_____

_____

Action	Days Needed	Target Dates: Begin	End	Employee

COMMITTEES, TASK FORCES, AND THE INFORMAL ORGANIZATION

"A camel is a horse created by a committee," goes an old saying. Whoever wrote that undoubtedly had a bad experience with committees. Your experience does not have to be the same.

Whether you call it a committee, task force, board, or commission, the function is the same. These bodies of individuals are delegated to consider, investigate or act on, or report on a matter of importance for the unit, department, or entire health care facility.

Using committees has several advantages over working alone or with one or two other people on an issue.

- They bring a greater amount of energy, experience, knowledge, and judgment to solving problems than can be offered by an individual working alone.

- They allow more efficiently coordinated plans and policies.

- They allow a smoother transmission of information.

- They promote cooperation among staff who are involved in committee work and their co-workers.

Nurse supervisors can make good use of committees. For example, you could recruit a Task Force to investigate and make recommendations regarding the implementation in your unit of a new state law requiring safety training. When a Task Force issues its recommendations, it disbands.

You could create a *Standing Committee,* too, that is a permanent fixture in your unit. For instance, Action Teams or Ad Hoc committees address such issues as work environment concerns (lack of break time for staff members, for example) or work-flow streamlining. These committees typically cross lines between job functions. They represent a cross-section of staff and are generally not led by nurse supervisors (although they may be formed at the urging of a nurse supervisor).

For committees to be successful, they must be formed with a clear purpose and authority. If the leadership and members are fuzzy about what they are doing, or if management won't give a committee's recommendations serious consideration, committees

- can become expensive in terms of time and money.

- may be forced to compromise to the point that their decisions are meaningless.

- a few powerful members may manipulate group so decisions made do not represent a consensus.

- may have difficulty coming to any decision at all.

As a nurse supervisor, you can help your committees avoid these pitfalls by following the guide-

lines you learned about planning and leading meetings. It will help you and the committee members if you review the purposes of the committee and the responsibilities of the members of the committee.

Whenever you work with groups of people, keep in mind that the formal organization is just the tip of the iceberg. Beneath the "official" committees, units, and divisions lies the *informal organization.*

The informal organization consists of the relationships among the formal organization's members. The power of the informal organization lies in its unwritten rules, or organizational norms. These unwritten rules come about through the pressures brought to bear by the relationships of co-workers. The unit "grapevine" is created by and maintained by the informal organization to cement the bonds between its staff members.

Be sure to recognize and take advantage of the informal organization. Remember that informal organizations bring their members feelings of belonging, status, and self-esteem.

SUPPLEMENTAL ACTIVITIES

1. The Action Planning Sheet is just one way of organizing a project. Two other popular methods are the PERT (Program Evaluation and Review Technique) Chart and the Milestone Chart. Research these two types of charts in the library and decide whether either of them might be useful to you now or in the future.

2. Meet with your boss or nurse supervisor and discuss the methods he or she uses to organize projects.

EXAM QUESTIONS

CHAPTER 7
Questions 55–62

55. Brenda decides to organize her approach to her daily load of mail. She decides to follow the method used in this course for dealing with paper. The method is

   a. HARD: Hang it on the bulletin board, Act on it, Route it, or Dump it.

   b. FAST: File it, Act on it, Send it on, or Throw it away.

   c. SOFT: Send it on, place it in the Out basket, File it, or Throw it away.

   d. TRASH: Throw it away, Route it upstairs, Act on it, Shuttle it.

56. The best way to ensure that you can supply accurate information about conversations or daily activities is to

   a. document the days' events.

   b. tape-record all conversations.

   c. enroll in a memory-improvement class.

   d. mentally review the day's events each night before you fall asleep.

57. Your options for dealing with each document that comes to you are to

   a. file it, act on it, send it on, or throw it away.

   b. file it, respond to it, or ask someone else to deal with it.

   c. place it in the out basket, file it, or throw it away.

   d. mark it for later action, keep it for information, or throw it away.

58. The first step in creating a weekly or a daily job plan is to

   a. set goals.

   b. rank the week's tasks.

   c. assign tasks.

   d. check your resources.

Questions 59–60 address the situation described in the paragraph below.

Ariana is a nurse supervisor who has been assigned the project of developing a plan for the more effective use of volunteers. One of the major tasks that volunteers help with is transporting patients to their cars after hospital discharge. Ariana is not familiar with the volunteer staff and how decisions are made about their utilization. She decides to find out as much as she can before taking action on it.

59. What should Ariana do first?

   a. Research equipment and supplies needed, volunteers needed and available, and any safety considerations.

   b. Set daily and weekly goals for the project and ask for her nurse supervisor's approval.

   c. Calculate the cost of the project to the health care facility and make a recommendation regarding it.

   d. Decide whether the project could mean a promotion for her and pass it on to others if not.

60. When Ariana's research is completed, what should be her next step?

    a. File her research where she can find it quickly when the need arises.

    b. Consult her nurse supervisor about the best staff nurses for the project team.

    c. Complete an action planning worksheet.

    d. Select a committee to set goals and deadlines.

61. One of the advantages of working with committees is that

    a. since committees are by nature democratic, people always get to voice their opinions in committees.

    b. most committees find it easier to come to decisions than do individuals working alone.

    c. they bring more energy and experience to problem solving than can be offered by an individual working alone.

    d. they are the most inexpensive option in terms of time and money.

62. One of the disadvantages of working with committees is that

    a. they make it more difficult to efficiently coordinate plans and information.

    b. they may have to compromise to the point that their decisions are meaningless.

    c. the transmission of information is more complicated when committees are involved.

    d. they tend to promote discord and lack of cooperation among staff nurses who serve on them.

CHAPTER 8

TIME MANAGEMENT FOR NURSE SUPERVISORS

INTRODUCTION

This chapter will give you a look at some time management principles that will help you keep your plans on track. You will have an opportunity to analyze how you spend your work day. You will learn how to recognize work that can be delegated and how to delegate it. Finally, you will learn about the seven rules of efficiency and the seven red flags that indicate a need for planning.

CHAPTER OBJECTIVE

After studying this chapter, you will be able to identify ways you can employ time management techniques to increase your effectiveness as a nurse supervisor.

LEARNING OBJECTIVES

Upon completion of this chapter, you will be able to:

1. Recognize typical "time-eaters."

2. Identify methods and benefits of delegating authority.

3. Recognize the seven rules of efficiency.

4. Choose situations that may indicate the need for planning.

LESSON CONTENT

Having a daily plan gives you a head start on managing your time. However, a typical workday can be full of unexpected events that require you to remain flexible. Good time management means having systems in place for dealing with the events you don't anticipate: Interruptions, crises, small problems, and unexpected paperwork.

TIME-EATERS

Time-eaters are the activities that keep you from accomplishing your primary objectives for the day. Socializing with your co-workers over a cup of coffee can be a time-eater or a necessary part of your day—everyone needs time to relax so that they will be more effective on the job. However, coffee breaks become time-eaters when they take priority over tasks that should have a higher priority. For instance, spending 45 minutes over coffee would be considered a time-eater.

Time-eaters fall into two categories: Those we generate ourselves, and those generated by our environment.

Self-Generated Time-Eaters

"We have met the enemy," said comic strip star Pogo, "and they is us." You can be your own worst enemy or your best friend when it comes to time-eaters. Look through the list of pitfalls below and see whether any of them apply to you.

Disorganization. If you spend 15 minutes searching for a paper or piece of equipment you had in your hands two days ago, chances are you need to review chapter 7 of this unit for hints on getting organized. Other areas that can eat your time include disorganized:

Work area. It should be organized so that you can easily reach frequently used supplies and equipment.

- Cabinets and shelves
- Desks
- Computers, printers, scanners and faxes
- Personal organizers
- Documents
- Layout of office

Procrastination. Many people find themselves procrastinating over small, boring, or unpleasant tasks. Try building in a reward—promise yourself a movie with a friend the night you finish that long report or an ice cream cone during your afternoon break if you get a certain task finished by then. You can even schedule your tasks in a sequence that rewards you—fun tasks following unpleasant ones. Make sure your rewards are immediate—they are more effective that way.

Lack of Interest in Work. If you find your work doesn't interest you, you may be burned out, or you may need to find ways to make your work more challenging. Burnout may require counseling with your boss, or talking with personnel about other job opportunities in the health care facility. To make your work more rewarding, review the suggestions under Procrastination (above). See if you can share your work or swap tasks with a co-worker, or ask your boss about additional training.

Perfectionism. You can paralyze yourself by requiring perfection of every task you complete. Give yourself permission to start out with a rough draft of whatever it is you're producing, and plan to revise it until it serves its purpose—not until it's perfect.

Environment-Generated Time-Eaters

Some of your time-eaters may seem to be beyond your control. While it may be true that you don't create the time-eaters on this list, it is also true that you are not at their mercy. In fact, these time-eaters are part of your job. Your schedule should be flexible enough to accommodate them.

Interruptions. Many nurse supervisors have an "open-door policy"—a practice of being available to staff at all times of the workday. Interruptions are the down side of an open-door policy. You may not want to revoke an open-door policy, if you have one. However, if interruptions are a problem for you, consider setting a two-hour "no interruptions" period when you take no calls and receive no visitors. Otherwise, try the suggestions listed below.

Visitors. Be polite but firm. When people drop in, stand up to greet them. Don't sit down, and don't invite them to sit. Discourage drop-ins by turning your desk away from the door.

Phone Calls. Some people actually set a timer near the telephone. When a business call turns social, they set the timer for three minutes. Even if you prefer not to use a timer, practice being polite and firm about getting off the telephone.

Crises. If your day seems to be a series of crises that only you can handle, you probably need to take another look at how well you delegate work (see "Delegating Authority" later in this chapter).

The Team Approach. Some nurse supervisors arrange with other nurse supervisors to cover for them when they're not available. Then they return the favor when another nurse supervisor needs the coverage.

Mail and e-mail. Respond to letters and electronic mail as quickly as possible, or hand them on to someone else who can respond to them. (Sometimes the only response that is needed is a quick, note.) Follow the FAST principle you learned in chapter 7: File, Act, Send on, Throw away. Abuse of e-mail and the Internet at work for personal business is common. Make sure you set an example, along with other supervisors, in your use of both e-mail and the Internet.

Waiting Time. Some waiting is unavoidable. Limit waiting when you have an appointment by showing up on time, then waiting only 15 minutes. Ask the secretary to call you when your party is ready to see you and go back to work. If you must wait, keep work with you so that you can make use of the time.

Unproductive Meetings. Make sure the meetings you call don't fall into this category by following the guidelines in chapter 4. When you must attend someone else's meeting, first make sure you have to be there. If so, arrive on time and participate responsibly—be a presence meeting leaders welcome, not one they have to contend with.

ACTIVITY

To help find the time-eaters that deprive you of your most valuable resource, keep a time log for a week.

1. Select a typical week (no vacations or holidays).

2. Make and photocopy a time log sheet.

3. Record your activities every half-hour. Be specific. Include names of visitors and what you talked about.

4. Comment on each activity in the space provided. Note whether you were interrupted, what problems you encountered in completing the activity, whether the activity went more quickly than usual, etc.

5. At the end of the day, add up the time spent in major activities (telephone calls, meetings, dictating letters, etc.). Write totals and other comments at the bottom of the Log.

When you have a week's worth of logs, analyze them using the following guidelines:

1. Determine which part of the day tends to be the most productive. Identify in what way it is productive (most telephone calls made, most tasks accomplished, etc.). Determine why it is the most productive part of the day (fewest interruptions, you have more energy at that time, work requirements increase during that time, etc.).

2. Determine which part of the day tends to be least productive. Determine why it is the least productive.

3. Identify your biggest time-eaters (interruptions, visitors, searching for documents, meetings, etc.).

4. Identify which tasks could be delegated.

5. Identify times when you allow "pleasure before work"—for example, chatting with staff nurses instead of drafting a memo.

6. Determine approximately what percentage of your work time is productive. Decide how you feel about this figure (shocked, pleased, embarrassed, etc.). Decide whether it should change and, if so, what it should be.

7. If you believe you need to improve your time management skills so that more of your time is productive, read a book on time management (the reference list at the end of the text is a good place to start). Develop objectives (for example, to increase productive time by 15%) and a plan for reaching them.

DELEGATING AUTHORITY

One of your most powerful time management tools is the delegation of your authority. Because no one person in an organization can do all its tasks, no one can exercise all the authority for making decisions. The number of people a nurse supervisor can efficiently supervise and make decisions for is limited. At some point, then, authority must be delegated. When nurse supervisors delegate well-defined tasks to staff, they can devote more time to activities such as planning.

A lack of delegation can decrease moral and staff initiative. Delegating authority can benefit the staff nurses in your unit. It can

- reward initiative.

- teach staff to do research and develop potential solutions.

- help create a sense of self-worth among staff nurses.

- give staff the opportunity to set their own goals.

Remember, your work as a nurse supervisor is rated on what your staff does, not on how much work you take on yourself. Being able to delegate authority is critical to your success as a nurse supervisor.

Planned Delegation

As you make the transition into a supervisory position, you'll gradually find that some tasks you'll want to delegate. You can delegate tasks that

- give others the opportunity to grow professionally or personally.

- are part of a new project.

- can be performed better by a subject matter expert in your unit.

- are relatively routine. Your job is governed by the principle of exception.

Only the unusual should be brought to you. Others can often handle routine work. This DOES NOT mean that you should delegate tasks you don't like because they are "routine." It does mean that tasks that are routine for you might be welcome challenges for someone else (Tappen, 1995).

When you have identified a task you wish to delegate, follow the steps below.

STEP 1 Choose one of your staff members to take over the task you've identified. To do this, review the qualifications, skills, and job descriptions of each of your staff members. Refer to some of the charts you made for chapter 7, and remember to match people to tasks.

STEP 2 Instruct the staff on how to perform the task and give feedback on the person's performance. Arrange training, if necessary. Explain the importance of the task to the operation of your work unit.

STEP 3 Leave the staff member alone to perform the task for a few days. Let the staff know you're available if problems arise.

STEP 4 Follow up. Praise the staff for work well-done. Arrange for more training if necessary. Consider using the four steps above to rotate tasks among staff. When staff members are thoroughly comfortable with each of their tasks, arrange for them to swap with each other. If possible, continue swapping tasks until everyone in your unit knows all the unit's jobs. Rotation provides a measure of security for the unit (a task won't be left undone because only one person knows how to do it), and helps prevent boredom. Rotation also provides a basis for comparing the productivity of each staff member against an average for all staff.

Joanne Bridges is the nurse manager of a Medical Ward. She has clinical lead nurses who work on each shift and seem eager to learn new tasks. Joanne would like all of these nurses to be familiar with processing the vacation requests through personnel and making up the monthly work schedule. She usually does this for all three shifts. Joanne decides to orient each clinical lead nurse to the procedure of processing vacation requests and have them make out the work schedules for the nurses on their shifts. For the first 3 months, Joanne reviews the schedules and vacation request slips. She finds the clinical lead nurses are enthusiastic about learning these new procedures.

An important concept to remember when delegating: You can delegate your authority, *but you can't delegate your responsibility for the results.* Make each decision to delegate carefully. How it is carried out will reflect on your abilities as a nurse supervisor.

Spontaneous Delegation

Some opportunities for delegating authority will come from your staff. Look at the following encounter.

Example

John Torres was on his way to an important nursing department meeting. Gloria Vick, one of his charge nurses, nearly ran into him hurrying around a corner.

"Oh, John," she said, "I'm so glad I caught you. We have a problem."

She quickly explained the problem and added, "I'm not sure what to do."

John glanced at his watch and saw that he had three minutes to get to the meeting.

"I'll look into it and let you know," John promised, striding off down the hall.

John made a couple of mistakes in this encounter. He allowed Gloria to assign him a responsibility, and he allowed her to consume part of one of his scarcest resources: His time.

John could have avoided the encounter entirely by training his staff not to rely on him so heavily for direction. Staff faced with on-the-job problems have three choices:

- Wait until the nurse supervisor tells them what to do.

- Ask the nurse supervisor what to do.

- Take action.

Unfortunately, staff often choose to wait or ask for further direction rather than act themselves. Why? Because their nurse supervisors, like John, don't encourage the initiative that delegation of authority can help create.

This is not to say that nurse supervisors actively discourage staff initiative. Rather, they take on problems that could have and should have been solved by the people who work for them. Like parents who always tie their five-year-old's shoes, these nurse supervisors rob their staff of opportunities to expand their abilities.

You leave your staff one choice—act—if you discourage them from waiting or asking for direction. While they may not have the authority to implement change, they can research problems and recommend solutions. Of course, you must take into consideration the experience and abilities of your staff before adopting such a policy.

To delegate authority to solve a problem, use one of two basic approaches: "Take care of it," or "Look into it."

"Take Care of It"

When you say, "Take care of it," you tell the staff member that you expect him/her to solve the problem. There are two variations on the Take Action approach: "Take care of it—no further contact with me is necessary," and "Take care of it and let me know what you did." Both approaches are to be used with staff members who can be trusted to accomplish the task without supervision.

"Look into It"

There are four variations of the "Look into it" approach:

- "Look into it and let me know what you intend to do; do it unless I say no."

- "Look into it and let me know what you intend to do; wait for my approval."

- "Look into it and let me know what alternative actions are available. List the pros and cons of each. Recommend one for my approval."

- "Look into it. Give me all the facts, and I'll decide what to do."

A policy of delegation can give staff a sense of belonging and makes their work more challenging and rewarding. It also makes your job easier and more challenging. Regardless of whichever policy you choose to adopt, make sure your staff know what your policy is.

THE SEVEN RULES OF EFFICIENCY

The efficient use of your time is governed by seven principles. They are:

RULE 1: Do your least-favorite tasks first. Don't let these jobs hang over you. Undone, they sap your energy and create low-level "worry static." Finished, they give you freedom to move on to more pleasant tasks with a clear conscience.

RULE 2: Touch paper once. For each letter, memo, or document you receive, MAKE A DECISION! One approach is the FAST system discussed in chapter 7.

RULE 3: Group similar tasks. This allows you to complete a number of tasks in a single sitting using the same resources and work area. You can group

- phone calls
- letter dictation
- report writing
- filing
- approving time sheets
- site visits (by geographical location)

RULE 4: Do regular housekeeping. Most papers filed away for a year or more are never used. Scheduling a regular "spring cleaning" of your files will make it possible for you to quickly find the piece of paper you need, when you need it. Use the same principle to deal with organizing, cleaning, and conditioning tools and equipment.

RULE 5: Work at a pace that feels right for you. For most people, a relaxed pace is best. They work steadily for a couple of hours at a time, then take a break to stretch, rest their eyes or sit down, then go back to work. Experiment with different pacing to find out what works for you. But remember—if you are exhausted at the end of every day or find yourself dreading the sound of the alarm each morning, you may need to reevaluate your work pace.

RULE 6: Eliminate "busy work." During slow times, people sometimes create little jobs or routines to take up the slack—"busy work." These little tasks can take on a life of their own, piling up and being carried on for years. Part of the nurse supervisor's job is to keep an eye out for busy work and eliminate it. When in doubt, ask yourself "Is this job really necessary?"

RULE 7: Eliminate perfectionism. Perfectionism is not the same thing as attention to quality.

For each task you set out to do, you need to set priorities. Decide what is the most important aspect of the job, the speed with which it must be accomplished and what its finished appearance is to be. Decide whether it is the most important task of the day or one of the least important.

SEVEN "RED FLAGS"

There are warning signs that let you know it's time to review your planning and organization. These red flags are

FLAG #1 Low production quality/quantity. This is the biggest red flag of all. It can be the result of any of the warning signs listed above; check them all.

FLAG #2 Noise. Not every health care environment can be pin-drop quiet. Some environments get noisy at certain times of the day. You are the best judge of how much noise is too much for your clients and your staff. When noise reaches unacceptable levels, check for orderly work flow, efficient layout and adequate work assignments.

FLAG #3 Piles of papers. Stacks of papers on benches or desks could mean you're not delegating enough work, lack of training, lopsided work assignment or an attempt to appear busy.

FLAG #4 Lopsided busy-to-idle ratio. When some workers are consistently busy while others are idle, you could be seeing the results of poor distribution of work, lack of training, or inadequate delegation.

FLAG #5 Bickering. When people argue a lot, you may find they don't understand the lines of authority or work procedures.

FLAG #6 Boredom or fatigue. When this red flag goes up, check to see whether your staff have adequate goals or incentives. Make sure there is enough work to do and that it is challenging enough. Also, check to see whether you've made a good match between the task and the worker.

FLAG #7 Shortages of supplies or equipment. Reviewing resources is the first step of planning. If you're short, figure out what went wrong. Review your planning procedures.

Some nurse supervisors keep the list of the seven red flags posted where they can see it as a reminder to keep their eyes open for ways to improve efficiency or make better use of their time.

SUPPLEMENTAL ACTIVITY

1. Make five copies of the following Daily Time Log. Keep a log for each day of the week for one week. Can you see a pattern in times of the day when you get very little accomplished? What is happening during those times? Are you spending more time performing some tasks than you thought? Use your log results to help you recognize "time-eaters" and devise a plan to help you deal with them.

DAILY TIME LOG

Day of Week: M   T   W   T   F   Date:

Time	Activity	Remarks
7:00		
7:30		
8:00		
8:30		
9:00		
9:30		
10:00		
10:30		
11:00		
11:30		
12:00		
12:30		
1:00		
1:30		
2:00		
2:30		
3:00		
3:30		
4:00		
4:30		
5:00		
5:30		

Was this day _____ Typical? _____ Busier than usual? _____ Slower than usual?

Comments:

EXAM QUESTIONS

CHAPTER 8
Questions 63–69

63. Disorganization, perfectionism, and procrastination are all examples of

    a. work crises.

    b. job burnout.

    c. environment-generated time-eaters.

    d. self-generated time-eaters.

Questions 64–66 refer to the paragraph below.

Maria is the clinical coordinator of a medical floor. She arrived at work at 7 a.m. Monday. She sat in on report and made sure things were running smoothly in the unit. After this, Maria wanted to get started on her week's paperwork. Her first task was to clean off her desk. By the time she finished that task, the mail had arrived, so she decided to get that out of the way. Halfway through the mail, she looked up and noticed it was time to leave for a nursing education meeting. She arrived at the meeting on time; it was late getting started. She visited with another nurse for 15 minutes until the meeting began. During a break an hour later, Maria's supervisor approached her. "I'm sorry Maria, I meant to tell you that you didn't need to attend the nursing education meeting. It is only for committee members."

64. Maria's biggest problem this morning was

    a. procrastination.

    b. self-generated time-eaters.

    c. environment-generated time-eaters.

    d. lack of work skills.

65. Maria identifies several tasks that have become routine for her. One option for dealing with these tasks is to

    a. delegate them to someone who would welcome the challenge.

    b. try to do them increasingly quickly.

    c. hire a new clerk to help her accomplish them.

    d. rewrite her job description to eliminate these tasks.

66. One of Maria's head nurses caught Maria on the way to a late lunch. "This report just came from admissions," she said, "and it requires some changes in our staff requirements for the night shift. What should I do?" If Maria is interested in the most efficient use of her time, what would be the best thing Maria could say to this lead nurse?

    a. "Put it in the in basket on my desk."

    b. "I'll take care of it right after lunch."

    c. "Lunch can wait. Let's talk about this now."

    d. "Take care of it and let me know what you did."

67. One of the benefits of delegating authority is that

    a. it allows nurse supervisors to unload boring, unpleasant, or routine tasks.

    b. it provides nurse supervisors with practice at giving direction.

    c. most tasks can be performed better by non-nurse supervisory staff members.

    d. it helps create a sense of self-worth among staff.

68. Alison is a clinical coordinator who enjoys making rounds to the units. However, she schedules checking on the resolution of yesterday's unanswered problems first. Which of the Seven Rules of Efficiency is she employing?

    a. do your least-favorite tasks first

    b. eliminate "busy work"

    c. group similar tasks

    d. touch paper once

69. Alison has had several complaints that the P.M. shift has extra time on their hands while the day shift staff is working overtime and not getting all their tasks completed. What is needed in this situation?

    a. more productive workers on the A.M. shift

    b. increased staffing on the day shift

    c. planning, to distribute the work more evenly

    d. nothing, this always happens

CHAPTER 9

GUIDING TEAM PROJECTS

INTRODUCTION

This chapter is divided into two parts corresponding to two main areas of supervisory responsibilities in regard to team projects.

Part One: Coordinating Team Projects

Part Two: Supporting Team Projects

Part One describes the planning and organizing activities that go into coordinating a team project. It also discusses methods for ensuring that team projects progress according to plan and that performance and quality standards are met. Part Two discusses the supervisor's role in encouraging teamwork and individual commitment to team goals and objectives.

CHAPTER OBJECTIVE

After studying this chapter, you will be able to identify ways to coordinate and support team efforts.

LEARNING OBJECTIVES

Upon completion of this chapter, you will be able to:

1. Recognize the functions of progress charts.

2. Identify methods for resolving team conflicts.

3. Identify methods for involving team members in a team project.

4. Specify one of the benefits of conflict.

5. Identify the functions of formal group meetings.

PART ONE— COORDINATING TEAM PROJECTS

Your staff will rely on you, their nurse supervisor, to lay the groundwork for smooth team operations by determining the scope of the work involved in a unit project and conveying that information to them in specific, concrete terms. How extensive is the task? Does management have a definite date by which it must be completed, or is it an ongoing process? How many nurses will be involved? Will there be other groups involved? You may need to sit down with your immediate supervisor to help you answer these and other questions.

When you have a pretty good idea of what kind of effort is required, you will need to do some careful planning and organization. You will need to

- identify available resources.

- determine standards of performance and quality.

- establish target dates.

- design a tracking system.

Each of these activities will be introduced here in the context of team coordination.

IDENTIFY AVAILABLE RESOURCES

One of your first planning priorities is to determine what resources you will need to achieve organizational goals and what resources you can realistically get your hands on. The kind of resources you need will depend upon the type of work involved and may include people, money, equipment, facilities, and supplies. If you know the job well, you may already know the kind of resources you require. However, if you are new at this, you may need to get some help from your immediate supervisor.

People are your most important resource. You will need to assess the type of talent you need, the level of skill required, and weigh those needs against the talent actually available to you. Some team members may be very experienced and others may have little experience. You may need to set up training to bring some members "up to speed." You may need to pair an experienced person with an inexperienced person. If you have only one experienced person, you may consider making this individual a team leader to assist you in monitoring the team. If none of your team members is experienced, you may need to arrange for technical experts to step in from time to time. These are all factors you must plan for in the very beginning, and your team members may have some valuable contributions to offer in this regard.

DETERMINE STANDARDS OF PERFORMANCE AND QUALITY

In this day of extremely high health care costs, all health care facilities need to be concerned with efficient service. Health care facilities must provide high-quality client care at the lowest possible cost. A commitment to quality health care increases the following:

- Client satisfaction.

- The organization's standing in the community.

- Pride within the organization.

Your team will look to you for guidance in achieving project goals. They will want to know the following:

- How much work needs to be done?

- How fast does the work need to be done?

- What are the minimum quality standards to be met?

As a nurse supervisor, you will need to answer these questions for the team. You will need to convey management's commitment to productivity and high-quality care by setting up standards that are realistic, that team members can understand, and that can be monitored as the project progresses.

Establish Target Dates

To start your nursing team off in the right direction, you will need to set up some initial target dates. If management has given you a definite completion date, this date will serve as your starting point. The experience of your nurses will determine how strong a role you take in setting intermediate target dates. If they are experienced, they will be able to help you a great deal in determining how long various tasks will take. Once a project has begun, even the inexperienced nurses will begin to get a more accurate idea of how long it takes to accomplish various tasks and will be able to participate in setting intermediate target dates.

IMPORTANT

Your nursing staff will work harder and more efficiently when they can target their efforts toward definite due dates. Your staff will have a greater commitment to meeting deadlines when they have a role in setting them.

Design a Tracking System

It is not enough to set up target dates and standards of performance and quality. You also need to set up a tracking system to determine whether the target dates, performance standards, and quality standards are met. Regular, informal meetings are an excellent way to keep on top of how the team is progressing. It is also helpful to have a visible, concrete way for the nursing team to track its progress, as demonstrated in the following chart.

NAME OF TASK	COMPLETED
Job #1	3/14/99
Job #2	5/22/99
Job #3	
Job #4	

For some of us, elementary school holds memories of how good it felt when the teacher gave us gold stars when we turned in assignments. The same type of system works for adults. A progress chart

- helps you, as nurse supervisor, monitor the nursing team's performance.

- involves the team members in monitoring their own progress.

- rewards productivity.

- provides incentive for continued progress.

ACTIVITY

Identify a job at home or at work that you have been putting off. Break the job down into smaller, concrete tasks. Then select a way of charting your progress (such as the sample chart shown in this lesson). Choose a method that will be rewarding for you. The idea is to make sure you see yourself making progress. It works best if you set up tasks that have a definite beginning and end. Your method won't work if you can't tell when a task is finished.

PULLING IT ALL TOGETHER

Once your planning is underway, you will need to act on the information you have accumulated by

- allocating time, money, materials, and facilities.

- making assignments based on team member functions and skills.

- arranging necessary training.

- coordinating activities among nursing team members and other groups.

Your team members can make important contributions to these activities. If you involve them as a team from the beginning, you will give the inexperienced nurses a taste for working with others toward the same goals, and you will give all nursing team members a greater commitment to the decisions that are made.

PART TWO— SUPPORTING TEAM PROJECTS

Bringing your staff together to assist you in initial planning and organizational activities is an excellent first step toward building an effective team from a group of individual staff members. Having taken this first step, your focus can turn to encouraging your team in their long-term projects to work cooperatively toward common goals and objectives.

There are three important ways you can support your nursing team's projects:

• Encourage open communication.

• Encourage team participation.

• Support team conflict resolution.

ENCOURAGE OPEN COMMUNICATION

All your nursing staff members who have an investment in the outcome of a project rely on you to keep them informed, and you rely on them to keep you informed. If you want to keep all interested parties working cooperatively, you will need to pay particular attention to keeping horizontal and vertical lines of communication open and functioning. This means finding out exactly who needs information from you, the kind of information they need, and the best way to provide the information. It also means finding out how and from whom you can get the information you need to keep team operations running smoothly.

Horizontal Communication

Horizontal communication refers to communication between you and your peers or groups of peers. If your project requires coordination with other teams, a free exchange of information among teams and nurse supervisors is essential to coordinating project activities and to maintaining cooperative relationships. Horizontal communication within nursing teams is also essential. Nurse team members need to exchange job information, ideas, and constructive information among themselves.

Vertical Communication

Vertical communications refers to communication between upper management, you, and those you supervise. You are the channel through which information flows from management to your team and back. If this flow is disrupted, management loses touch with the work (whether goals are being achieved within defined deadlines or of any real-life situations that may be interfering with the achievement of these goals). Your team may lose touch with what management is expecting and may stray from meeting its obligations. Your nursing team needs to know right away when there are directives from management, changes in priorities or target dates, or new guidelines to implement. Keeping your team informed will minimize confusion, misinformation, and rumors.

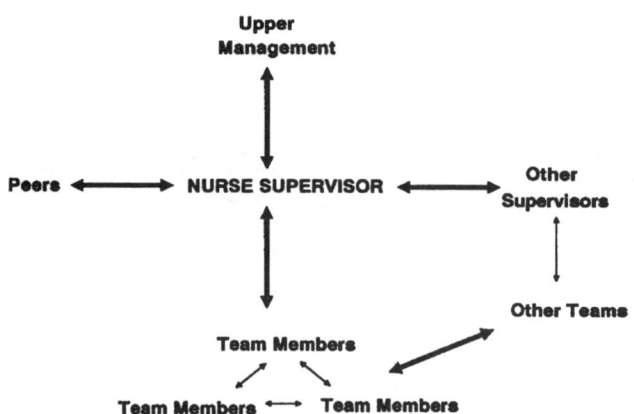

VERTICAL AND HORIZONTAL COMMUNICATION

Methods of Transmitting Information

There are several ways to keep your nurses informed. You may find yourself using all of them. Methods for transmitting information include:

- Progress reports.
- Formal and informal group meetings.
- Individual meetings.
- Memos.

Progress Reports

Your boss may want to receive information from you through verbal reports, written reports, or both. Progress reports are commonly used to communicate with management and are usually submitted on a weekly or monthly basis. The progress report tells management:

- What has been accomplished during a specific time period.
- What still needs to be accomplished.
- Problems or obstacles that have been encountered.
- The impact of problems or obstacles on deadlines.

Sometimes progress reports are shared with the team so the members can get an overall view of the project or job.

Formal and Informal Group Meetings

Group meetings are used when you want several people to receive the same information at the same time and when you want people to provide input on the issues involved.

Group meetings can be formal or informal. Informal meetings are very useful on an impromptu basis, when your nursing team needs to work out immediate concerns or when you want to pass on a compliment about their work. When you have informal meetings with your team members, you need to make sure all team members are included so that everyone has a chance to absorb the information.

Formal meetings also serve some important functions. They provide an excellent opportunity for your team to regroup when it has temporarily lost its focus. Formal meetings provide a chance to

- restate goals.
- make major adjustments in tasks, assignments, and target dates, when necessary.
- convey official feedback on the team's performance.

When you convene a formal meeting, it is important to prepare an agenda to get everyone on the same track. It is also important to document the meeting and distribute official meeting notes afterward to reinforce what was decided.

Individual Meetings. Sometimes individual team members want to discuss issues that do not concern other members of the team, or they may be reluctant to discuss certain issues in a group setting. In circumstances such as these, individual meetings are appropriate. In individual meetings, you can

- discuss issues not appropriate in a group setting.
- provide feedback on individual performance.
- find out if the individual's needs are being met within the group.

It is important in individual meetings not to draw energy away from the group process. In other words, don't try to address issues with the individual that the whole team should be addressing among themselves.

Example

Dan has been having difficulty concentrating lately. He and his wife are having marital problems. They have been seeing a counselor once a week, but they still frequently stay up late having arguments.

The project Dan is working on is the development of a job aid to place in the treatment room. This job aid will help staff recall the steps in conducting a neurological examination when assessing their patients. Dan was supposed to have an idea drafted for the layout of the job aid. Dan knows that the team has a deadline in two days, and he is afraid that his part of the job will not be done on time. Because this is a personal matter, Dan decides to discuss it privately with his supervisor.

Although Dan's lack of productivity may affect the team's ability to meet the next deadline, it is very appropriate for Dan to discuss the matter with his nurse supervisor alone. Not only does it involve Dan's personal life, but his nurse supervisor will be responsible for helping the team find ways to take over some of Dan's responsibilities or to adjust the deadline until Dan can devote his full attention to the project.

Memos. Memos are important communication tools when you want to

- document an important directive or change.

- ensure that everyone gets the same information.

- reinforce what you have stated verbally.

- maintain a written history of project directives.

Example

DATE:	3/5/96
TO:	Team Members
FROM:	Jill Morris, RN OB-GYN Supervisor
SUBJECT:	Change in CPR Instructor Certification Target Date

This will confirm that the target date for all practical and classroom work to be completed for CPR Instructor Certification has been extended from March 31 to April 30, 1996. Additional classes to complete the practical portion of the class will be held once a week in Continuing Education Room 320. See the extended schedule posted on the Nursing Education Bulletin Board.

If you have any questions or suggestions, please contact me.

Memos are a rather impersonal way of communicating. Make sure you don't use them as a substitute for talking to your team.

ACTIVITY

On a separate sheet of paper, list all of the ways your supervisor communicates with you. Then note the kind of information your supervisor provides in each type of communication. Does your supervisor use any methods of communication that are not covered in this lesson?

ENCOURAGE TEAM PARTICIPATION

Building an effective, productive team from a group of individuals is a definite challenge for any nurse supervisor, particularly a new nurse supervisor. Not only are you likely to have nurses with different skill and experience levels, you will also have people of different

- ages.

- sexes.

- races.

- cultural backgrounds.

- educational backgrounds.

You will have staff members with different personalities, values, and habits. And, you will have people who naturally work well with others and those who prefer working independently.

Getting all of these individuals to work together toward a common goal requires commitment from you. You will need to declare both in words and in actions that you support organizational goals. And you will need to make it clear that you and management

- value the fresh ideas and new perspectives that individual differences can bring to the team.

- look positively at those individuals who demonstrate willingness to work cooperatively with others.

- value an atmosphere of mutual support.

Finally, you will need to remind your staff that you cannot achieve organizational goals without the involvement of everyone.

Encourage Individual Participation

Unless all the nursing staff on the team are contributing members, the team will not function at its full capability. A single noncontributing individual can decrease the productivity of the entire team.

You can encourage individual participation by conveying the sincere impression that you need the help of every staff member in accomplishing the departmental goals. To convince your staff that you value their input, you need to

- encourage members to express their ideas.

- help people feel good about their own talents and skills.

- respect individual differences.

- give periodic praise for meeting job requirements.

- praise teamwork, but also recognize individual contributions.

- guide and encourage personal growth.

ACTIVITY

Mike is a shy, reserved person. Whenever he is given an assignment, he quietly sets out to work on it. He always finishes promptly and does very well in accomplishing his portion of the assignment.

Mike has been assigned to a new project. He will be working with four other nurses in the hospital. Although the new assignment is a challenge, Mike is worried about having to coordinate his work with others. Also, he doesn't feel comfortable speaking in front of a group of people.

Assume you are Mike's nurse supervisor. On a separate sheet of paper, list the things you would do to encourage him to participate in this team effort.

As you may have realized, there is no single right response. Here are some suggestions.

1. At the first meeting, when you are introducing the team members, you could introduce Mike as someone whose hard work and good ideas are noticed and appreciated. In this way, you will be helping Mike feel good about himself and will be pointing out to the other team members what is valuable about Mike.

2. You could sit down with Mike individually. Point out areas in which he has particular talents. Ask him if he will offer some suggestions in these areas during the next team meeting.

3. Another way to encourage Mike to participate would be to reinforce the behaviors you want him to exhibit. For instance, when he does speak up in a team meeting, give him your full attention and his suggestions your full consideration. Once Mike sees that others do value what he has to say, he may begin to participate more actively. He may never be as good a leader as his fellow team member, Elizabeth, but he has talents to offer that Elizabeth doesn't.

Encourage Mutual Support

You need to know you can depend on your team, your team needs to know it can depend on you, and team members need to know they can depend on one another. In order for an environment of mutual support to exist, your staff needs to know that you will:

- Share control, responsibilities, and credit with them.

- Be consistently honest in your interactions with them.

- Maintain individual and group contact to see how things are going.

- Stand up for them with management.

Example

Marsha Harris devised a flow sheet for shift report she believed would help nurses organize their notes and remember to cover all the essential information. She took the idea to her nurse supervisor. The supervisor didn't want to build up Marsha's hopes, but she suggested Marsha submit the flow sheet to be implemented throughout the entire medical facility.

When her supervisor told management about Marsha's idea, they were enthusiastic and decided to give it a trial run. The flow sheet was a success. Marsha's supervisor made sure that management and everyone else in the department knew that it was Marsha's idea. When Marsha's co-workers saw the commendation Marsha received, they began to think of ways they could help unit routines run more smoothly.

In this example, Marsha's nurse supervisor had the right idea. She knew how important it is to encourage initiative, even if every idea isn't a "winner."

Once an environment of mutual support is established, you will need to check your own behavior periodically to make sure you don't undermine your team's confidence. Make sure you really are sharing control and responsibilities with your team members and are not using their inexperience or lack of skills as an excuse for doing the work yourself. Also, be sure to:

- Keep regular contact with your team members (but not to the extent that you are hanging over their shoulders).

- Provide constructive feedback.

- Avoid being overly critical.

- Get essential information to your team members so that they can perform their jobs successfully.

When people work as a team in a mutually supportive environment, they soon discover the benefits of helping one another. Team members see the effect their projects and those of their colleagues have on client care. They find themselves reaching higher levels of accomplishment. Members gain confidence in their own ideas when they know others share their views and are acting in harmony with them. Working together leads to and reinforces their commitment to support one another and to accomplish organizational goals.

SUPPORT POSITIVE CONFLICT RESOLUTION

Whether we like to admit it or not, conflict is normal when people are working closely together (Sullivan, 1994). Staff members have different motivations, different values, different working styles, different ways of expressing themselves, and different levels of tolerance.

ACTIVITY

Doug Fitzpatrick and Sue Yang are patient educators on the same project team. They have separate assignments, but Sue's assignment cannot be completed until Doug completes the first part of his assignment.

Sue always appears extremely busy. Her desk is always stacked with papers, and she takes work home almost every night. She never misses a deadline. However, it is very difficult to have a conversation with her because she never has the time.

Doug takes a more relaxed attitude toward life. His work is usually out on time, but he feels no need to hustle and rarely stays after hours to finish an assignment. Doug's co-workers like him because he always takes the time to listen to what they have to say.

On a separate sheet of paper, briefly describe the potential conflicts you see between Sue and Doug.

If you pointed out that Doug and Sue may find themselves in a conflict over their different styles of working, you were right. The conflict probably wouldn't surface as an issue over working styles.

However, any conflicts Doug and Sue may have are likely to have this basic issue as the cause. Another potential conflict is Sue's dependence on Doug finishing his work on time.

Benefits of Conflict

Your response and the responses of the team members determine whether the results of conflict are positive or negative. When conflict is avoided or approached on a win/lose basis, hostilities will develop, communications will break down, and trust and mutual respect will deteriorate. However, conflict can stimulate growth and creativity when people use it as an opportunity to explore new ideas, learn about the values of others, and test their problem-solving capabilities.

Responses to Conflict

People have various ways of dealing with conflict, just as they do with other kinds of stress. The advantages and disadvantages of different responses to conflict are summarized in the table that follows.

Although the responses shown in the table below can be effective depending on the type and magnitude of the conflict, problem-solving is a more constructive approach that may be used in a variety of circumstances.

Responses to Conflict	Advantages	Disadvantages
Avoidance	It can be used successfully when conflicts are minor and not worth the time and effort	When some conflicts are ignored or denied, they tend to grow bigger and more serious.
Confrontation	Gets conflict out in the open where it can be looked at and discussed	It can be very offensive and may cause less-aggressive team members to withdraw and not participate.
Concession (Giving In)	It is cooperative behavior and can be used in the same situations as avoidance (the situation is not worth the discomfort of bringing it up).	Team members may use this approach to promote group cooperation at the expense of their own opinions and values.
Compromise (Mutual Agreement)	It acknowledges the right of individuals to disagree with one another. All parties gain some of what they want.	Individuals often settle for less than they want in the interest of the common good.
Win-Win	Everybody gets the **main** things they want.	It takes the most time.

The Problem-Solving Approach to Conflict

A problem-solving approach minimizes the anxiety and stress that accompany a conflict because it forces people to look at issues less emotionally. It is a fact-gathering approach that

- separates the problem from the people by focusing on the issues behind the conflict rather than on the conflict itself.

- separates what can be done from what cannot be done.

- states the problem in more realistic language.

- concentrates on outcomes instead of individual opinions or positions.

- reaffirms team priorities.

When a team uses the problem-solving approach, no attempt is made to "win" at someone else's expense, as is often the motive in the confrontational response. All team members have a voice in the process, and individual needs and positions are respected. Although there may be some concessions and compromises involved, the solutions reached are based on a thorough examination of the facts and on what will best accomplish team goals and objectives.

ACTIVITY

Victoria, the team leader, has come to you for advice. The team has strayed from the quality standards that you all agreed on in the beginning of the project. Doug blames Ralph. He says that Ralph doesn't pay enough attention to details and that the rest of the team has just picked up Ralph's bad habits. Victoria feels at a loss because an argument between Doug and Ralph has been brewing for some time. Everyone on the team has taken sides in the dispute, and it is interfering with the team's productivity.

On a separate piece of paper, briefly describe how you would handle this conflict.

Check your suggestions against the conflict resolution system described below.

Your Role in Resolving Team Conflict

Your role as a nurse supervisor is to provide a flexible, positive environment in which conflicts are minimal and easily resolved. It is not to step in every time there is a problem. You can support your team by

- teaching your team members to understand conflict and resolve it constructively with stress management and problem-solving techniques.

- negotiating a solution only if it looks like the conflict is getting out of control.

IMPORTANT

People are much more likely to be satisfied with solutions to conflicts if they've had a part in developing the solutions.

In the conflict between Ralph and Doug it appears that only avoidance and confrontation have been used to respond to the conflict. To determine if you should step in at this point, you need to find out if Victoria and the team have tried the problem-solving approach.

If the team has not tried the problem-solving approach, it would probably be best to place responsibility for solving the conflict back in the hands of the team with the suggestion that they take the time to try the fact-gathering approach.

If the team has already tried the problem-solving approach and cannot seem to get beyond the personal issues, you probably should offer your assistance. Using the problem-solving approach to resolve conflicts takes some practice, and inexperienced teams may need your help the first time they try it. If you have to step in, it is important for you to remember not to take responsibility away from the team for solving the conflict.

You should try to limit your role to:

- Asking questions to open the discussion.

- Listening and summarizing both feelings and facts.

- Shifting the team's attention from individual positions in the dispute to what needs to be accomplished.

- Reaffirming team priorities.

Using the problem-solving approach, the team should be able to identify two separate issues:

1. The conflict between Doug and Ralph.

2. The team deviation from quality control standards.

Issue #1: Due to its sensitive nature and to the ongoing impact their dispute is having on team productivity, you may need to set up an individual meeting with Doug and Ralph to explore the reasons behind their conflict and ask for their help in finding a solution.

Issue #2: After taking a close, careful look at the quality control issue, the team may find that

- the quality control standards no longer fit the type of work they are doing and need to be updated, **OR**

- the team has temporarily lost its focus and needs to get back to its real work.

If you and the team working together cannot find a suitable solution to either issue and the conflict continues to escalate, you may need to seek outside help from someone with a fresh and objective viewpoint.

The degree to which a team requires nurse supervisory intervention depends on the type of job, the skills of the individual team members, and on the effectiveness with which the team members learn to work together. When you are a nurse supervisor, you may want to make it one of your priorities to create a team that functions with minimal supervision. Your role with a self-sufficient team could be limited to securing resources, establishing guidelines, keeping lines of communication open and functioning, and supporting the team's progress along the established guidelines.

EXAM QUESTIONS

CHAPTER 9
Questions 70–74

70. Progress charts serve several functions. Some of those functions are to

    a. discipline those who don't perform and reward those who do.

    b. keep track of the number of team meetings held per week and keep people busy.

    c. reward productivity, provide incentive, and monitor team's progress.

    d. show the team members what happens when people don't do what they're supposed to do.

71. What is one of the functions of formal group meetings?

    a. Provide feedback on individual performance.

    b. Restate goals when the team has lost focus.

    c. Resolve team member conflicts.

    d. Find out if individual needs are being met.

72. To convey the impression that you value your nursing staff's input, you should

    a. encourage staff members to express their ideas.

    b. hold as many meetings as possible.

    c. issue memos whenever policies change.

    d. try to get raises for your staff nurses.

73. One of the benefits of conflict is

    a. it lets you know where everyone stands.

    b. it can stimulate growth and creativity.

    c. it shows you who the winners and the losers are in your work unit.

    d. it makes work more interesting.

74. Susan was appointed to direct a project team of six staff nurses. Two of Susan's team members are fighting over project deadlines. Susan thinks the conflict is probably a personality problem, and waits to see if the two can work out their differences. Finally, one of the two asks Susan for help. What should Susan's response be?

    a. "No way! You people solve this yourself."

    b. "Have you two tried problem-solving techniques yet?"

    c. "I will decide by tomorrow at 2 p.m. My decision is final."

    d. "Which one of you would like to be transferred?"

CHAPTER 10

INTERVIEWING AND ORIENTING NURSES

INTRODUCTION

In this section, you'll examine the nurse supervisor's role in the hiring process and the orientation of new staff members. You'll learn the basic steps in the interviewing process, how to plan an interview and how to choose the best candidate. You'll also learn the importance of sticking to objective questions during an interview and how to make sure that your questions are objective. You'll learn how to make new staff feel at home once you've hired them and how to make sure the newcomer gets all the information he or she needs to get through the first few days on the job.

CHAPTER OBJECTIVES

After studying this chapter, you will be able to identify skills needed for interviewing and orienting new nurses to your workplace.

LEARNING OBJECTIVES

Upon completion of this chapter, you will be able to:

1. Identify the two most important factors to consider when evaluating the best candidate for the job.

2. Distinguish between appropriate and inappropriate interview questions.

3. Recognize questions you should ask yourself when analyzing a vacant position.

4. Recognize appropriate ways to introduce a new staff member to the job, the health care facility, the people and the procedures.

5. Identify characteristics of the interview process which uphold the Civil Rights Act.

LESSON CONTENT

Choosing, orienting, and training new staff nurses are important duties. Close attention to these tasks can help ensure

- better client care.
- lower turnover.
- lower hiring costs.
- shorter staff adjustment periods.
- fewer complaints.
- fewer disciplinary problems.
- higher morale.
- better safety records.
- less waste of materials.

INITIAL SCREENING OF JOB APPLICANTS

Most of the work in obtaining new nursing staff is usually done by a health care facility's Department of Human Resources (DHR) and the Nurse Recruiter. Applicants are recruited and screened for a vacant position through written public announcements. Many announcements are in classified advertising in local newspapers and may be vague about the eligibility requirements for the position.

Applicants for nursing positions are screened by both the Nurse Recruiter and the DHR against the minimum requirements. After initial screenings, first-level managers and supervisors collaborate to select the best person for each position.

THE INTERVIEWING PROCESS

If there is one word that characterizes the interview process, it is objectivity. The purpose of the interview is to determine how well candidates will meet the demands of the positions for which they have applied, based upon their experience and skills. No subjective opinions, prejudices, biases, or preconceptions of "ideal" stereotypes may be a part of this process.

Also, what you perceive as a candidate's attitude should have no bearing on how you evaluate that individual's skills. For instance, you may think that a candidate who answers your questions more slowly than you would like is being rude or is slow-witted. You could be wrong—perhaps this person likes to think answers through before speaking. In any case, a person who answers slowly is not necessarily less capable of the work than someone who responds quickly.

This objectivity is mandated by Title VII of the Civil Rights Act, among other legislation and court decisions, and is known as Equal Employment Opportunity.

The interviewing process is made up of three phases.

Phase One: **Planning the Interview**

If you are conducting an interview or participating in an interview panel, prepare a written format, following this procedure:

STEP 1 **Analyze the vacant position.** Using the vacancy announcement as a reference, ask yourself these questions:

- What duties does the job include?
- Which duties are the most important?
- What skills and knowledge are necessary to perform the job?

STEP 2 **Prepare interview questions and model answers.** Your questions should give you the factual, job-related information you will need to evaluate the candidate's ability to do the work. They should include

- at least one lead question for each major area of the job. For example, "When did you first start caring for patients with COPD?"
- follow-up questions to explore major job responsibilities in detail. Follow-up questions to the lead question above might be:

  — "What types of ventilators did you work with?"

  — "Which one are you most comfortable with?"

  — "Tell me about your experiences with patients with permanent tracheostomies."

  — "Tell me about your experiences with assisting with endotracheal intubations."

  — "What do you enjoy most about working with COPD patients?"

You should use the same lead questions for every candidate you interview. However, follow-up questions will vary depending on each candidate's answers to the lead questions.

Your questions should:

Explore the candidate's experience. What the candidates can do and how well they do it is more important than how long they did it.

Explore the candidate's achievements. What is this person most proud of? What changes or innovations did the candidate bring about in a past job?

Explore job-related educational experiences. These can include nursing school, universities or colleges, vocation/technical school, military, continuing education and special training, etc.

Give candidates an opportunity to explain their qualifications. Ask candidates to elaborate on their knowledge or skills that relate to the position, especially if you feel a candidate lacks one of the essential qualifications.

You can ask DHR to send you a copy of each candidate's original application to help you prepare or ask the candidates to bring it or a resume with them to the interview. Remember, though—you must request applications for all of the candidates, not just one or two.

When you prepare interview questions, consult with the person who has that job now. See the table "Typical Interview Question Topics" at the end of this chapter for information on formulating appropriate and legal questions. Some health care facilities ask that you submit your questions to your Personnel Officer for review.

When you have completed your questions, write answers for them—the kind of answers you'd like to hear during the interviews. Use these answers to evaluate the candidate's responses. You can prepare the questions and model answers in a checklist format to reduce writing during the interview.

You might also consider including performance tasks; i.e., asking candidates to perform one or more tasks typical of the job. For example, asking a nurse to calculate a medication dosage.

STEP 3 **Schedule a time and place for each interview.** (If someone else has already scheduled a time and place, be sure to enter them on your calendar.) You will be responsible for final scheduling of when and where the interview takes place. Decide how much time you'll need for each interview. Allow equal time for each job candidate.

STEP 4 **Form an interview team.** (Sometimes, others accomplish this task.) Two or three evaluations are better than one. Be sure each panel member participates. Clarify roles and the selection process before the interviews.

STEP 5 **Get excited!** If you are in a positive frame of mind for each interview, you'll find the interviews will go more smoothly. Why is your attitude so important? Think about your own experiences as a job candidate in interviews. If you're like most people, the interviewer's attitude probably determined how comfortable you were during the interview. It may have even affected your attitude toward the job and the company itself. An interested, cheerful interviewer makes it easier for job candidates to answer questions about themselves and to think of their skills and experience for the job they're applying for.

Phase Two: **Conducting the Interview**

Keep the following guidelines in mind when interviewing.

• **Put the candidate and yourself at ease before you begin the interview.** Use your best manners—as if you were the one hoping to make a good impression (you are!). Introduce yourself. Smile. Shake hands. Use the candidate's name. Don't barricade yourself behind your desk. Make small talk for a few minutes, then describe how the interview will proceed and how long it will take. Encourage the candidate to ask questions throughout the interview.

- **Use appropriate questioning techniques.**

- **Use a friendly tone of voice.** Don't cross-examine or act suspicious.

- **Use open-ended questions.** Questions starting with what, why, how, or tell me encourage the candidate to share information. Questions starting with did you, will you, have you, or are you, can be answered with a flat yes or no.

- **Make your questions clear and understandable.** Stay away from jargon, technical phrases, and big words.

- **Use good listening skills.** Don't interrupt. Periodically summarize or restate the candidate's comments. Avoid showing disapproval or approval of the candidate's answers or comments. Allow yourself to be questioned.

- **Be direct.** Trick questions or leading questions are inappropriate and probably won't get you the information you need.

- **Stick to the guidelines for legal, job-related questions.**

- **Give the facts.** Not only are you interviewing the candidates, the candidates are interviewing the health care facility. Give candidates the information they need to make a decision about the job, and encourage questions. Topics to discuss include

  - salary and wage plans.

  - working conditions.

  - job descriptions.

  - promotional policies.

  - hospital policies or programs that are new

or have been recently improved (for example employee ergonomics programs or workplace violence training).

- employee benefits.

- working hours and time off.

- opportunities for in-service and continuing education.

- evaluation procedures.

- standards of nursing care adopted by the facility.

- methods used for delivery of client care.

- **Take notes.** Tell the candidate you will be taking notes during the interview.

These will help you make a hiring decision later. Notes also provide documentation in case of a discrimination complaint later. Put quote marks around any notes in which you quote the candidate. A brief checklist can keep notes to a minimum and still document information you need.

Write yourself a few brief notes on Post-it Notes after the candidate leaves—something that strikes you about the person—to help you recall this particular person later. Remember to remove the Post-it Notes later.

- **Conclude the interview and tour the unit.** When you feel you've collected all the information you need, ask if the candidate has anything to add or any questions to ask. Then, make time to tour candidates through the unit where they might work. This will help you gauge their comfort level. See if they ask appropriate questions about the unit. If you will not be the their immediate supervisor, make sure candidates meet this person so a bond can be formed between them. Then, if candidates are offered positions and accept them, they have made a commitment to both the job and their supervisors.

Let the candidate know when and how the

health care facility will be in contact regarding the result of the application and interviews. If a reference check or some other time-consuming process must be completed before the candidate is contacted, explain this and estimate the amount of time it will take. Give the candidate your telephone number. Avoid promises or hints. Say "thank you" and show the candidate out.

- **Let candidates know by telephone or mail where they stand.** Don't leave job candidates hanging. Let them know whether the process is taking longer than you expected, someone else was hired, or hiring has been delayed due to funding cuts.

ACTIVITY

Lisa is interviewing Roy for a job opening. They walk into the room and Lisa immediately sits down. Lisa asks him to tell her about his previous job experience that's related to the current job; Lisa writes down Roy's reply. Lisa also asks Roy what he has accomplished that he's most proud of. Next she asks him where he lived in the 1950s and writes down his answer. Then Lisa thanks Roy for coming to the interview.

- How did Lisa do?

- Did she miss any steps?

- Should she change anything?

- Did she do anything right?

- What did Lisa do well?

- What should she change?

Prepare your response before looking at the activity feedback.

Activity Feedback

Did well: Asked about previous applicable job experience and accomplishment he's proud of.

Do differently: Ask him to sit down. Do not ask where he lived. (It's not relevant to the job.) Ask if he has any questions. Tell him about the job. Tell him when he can expect a decision.

Equal Opportunity and Interview Questions. Your interview questions should never imply that one candidate might be favored over another for any reason other than job qualifications. Based on this guideline alone, many questions are clearly inappropriate. Others, however, are subtler.

Take this example: "The job requires that you may have to work night shifts occasionally, Ms. Smith. How will you provide for the care of your children?" This is not a job-related question. A person's child-care arrangements have nothing to do with his or her ability to do the work. Furthermore, this kind of question historically has been asked of women only; as such, it may be discriminatory.

How can you be sure a job candidate can handle late night shifts? Easy. Just ask: "How available are you to work the late night shift?"

Following is a chart of acceptable and unacceptable questions for typical interview topics.

Appropriate interview questions explore

- the candidate's experience.

- the candidate's achievements.

- the candidate's job-related educational experiences.

- Conviction Records. Candidates' criminal conviction records may be relevant to their suitability for a job. For example, a person with a child molestation conviction would not be the best choice for a job on the pediatrics ward. Candidates may be required to fill out and show the health care facility a conviction

TYPICAL INTERVIEW QUESTION TOPICS

TOPIC	ACCEPTABLE	UNACCEPTABLE
AGE	"If hired, you may have to show that your age meets legal requirements for this job."	"Are you under 70 years of age?" Any question that identifies candidates 40 to 65 years of age violates the Age Discrimination in Employment Act.
ARRESTS	None.	"Have you ever been arrested?"
CHILDREN	None.	"Do you have children under 18?" "How many children do you have?" "What arrangements do you have for the care of your minor children?" "Oh, you have kids? I have a three-year-old and six-year-old twins! How old are yours?"
CITIZENSHIP	"If hired, you may have to show proof of U.S. citizenship."	"Are you a U.S. citizen?" "Are you naturalized or native-born?" "Are your parents U.S. citizens?" "Are your parents naturalized or native-born?" "When did you acquire U.S. citizenship?" "Is your spouse a U.S. citizen?" "How long has your spouse been a U.S. citizen?" "May I see your naturalization papers?"
EDUCATION	"Where did you go to college?" "Have you attended any post-graduate courses?"	"When did you go to college?"
WORK EXPERIENCE	"Tell me about the work experience you've had that relates to this job." "Tell me about your experience in the U.S. Navy that relates to this job."	"Tell me about your military experience." "What type of military discharge did you receive?" "Were you ever reduced in rank?"
FRIENDS AND RELATIVES	None.	"Do you have any friends or relatives working for us?"
HEIGHT AND WEIGHT	(Unless directly related to a job requirement, questions about height and weight are unacceptable.)	"What's your weight?" "How tall are you?"
MARITAL STATUS	None.	"Are you married? Divorced? Separated? Widowed? Never married?" "What is your maiden name?" "Do you have a prior married name?" "What is your spouse's name?" "What does your spouse do for a living?"
ORGANIZATIONS	"What professional organizations do you belong to?" "Do you belong to any general community service organizations?" (No questions about organizations whose names indicate the race, religion, creed, national origin, or ancestry of its members.)	"Tell me about all organizations, clubs, societies, and lodges to which you belong."
PHOTOGRAPH	"If hired, you may be required to have a photograph taken."	"We like to have a photograph for our file. Did you bring one today?"

TYPICAL INTERVIEW QUESTION TOPICS

TOPIC	ACCEPTABLE	UNACCEPTABLE
PHYSICAL CONDITION	"If you are offered this job, it would be contingent upon your passing a physical exam."	"Do you have any physical disabilities?" "Are you being treated for any medical condition?" "Are you in good health?" "Have you ever received Worker's Compensation?"
RACE OR COLOR	None.	"Would you say your complexion is olive?" "What is that last name—Italian?" "Are you Chinese or Japanese?"
RELIGION	None.	"What is your religion?" "Would your religion prevent you from working Saturdays?" "Do you expect to get religious holidays off?"
CONVICTIONS	"Our appointing authority has asked for a conviction record form from each candidate. Did you bring it today?"	"Have you ever been convicted of a crime?" "Have you ever been in jail?"
CREDIT RECORD/FINANCIAL STATUS	(All questions about credit records and financial status are probably unlawful unless required by business necessity.)	"How is your credit record?" "Do you have any debts?" "Do you own your own home?" "Do you own your own furniture? Car?" "Have you ever been refused a fidelity bond?" "Have your wages ever been garnisheed?" "Have you ever received unemployment compensation?"

record form. Requesting candidate conviction information is at the option of the health care facility. However, if such information is requested from one candidate, it should be requested from all candidates to avoid discriminatory treatment.

Confidentiality is also a concern. Return the conviction record form to the candidate at the end of the interview.

Phase Three: Recommending the Best Person for the Job

Nurse supervisors participating in the selection process are asked for their recommendations. Your job is to choose objectively, based on the candidate's application and interview, and any applicable exam results. The best way to accomplish this is to evaluate each candidate on paper. Your recommen-

dations are contingent upon the candidate meeting any requirements by your health care facility for a physical exam, a polygraph, drug and alcohol testing, background checks, or legal right to work in the United States.

A form like the one that follows can help in evaluating candidates. Each candidate's initials go in one of the boxes under "CANDIDATES." Knowledge, skills, and education blanks are filled out based on the job description as it appeared in the vacancy announcement. Each candidate is ranked according to the three-point ranking at the top of the page. The ranking is entered in the appropriate space. The numbers are totaled at the bottom.

Sometimes, the totals are different enough that the choice is clear. When two or more candidates' scores are close, the choice is not so easy. In that case, look at the strengths and limitations of each candidate and ask yourself:

• How well do these strengths match the requirements of the job?

• How important are these limitations to the performance of this job?

The best candidate is the person with the best **job-related** pattern of critical strengths and the fewest **serious** limitations.

ORIENTATION

A new staff member's first day is the most important one on the calendar. The impressions the newcomer receives (whether the individual is new to the health care facility or transferring from another unit) will stay with the staff member for a long time to come. A warm and thorough welcome can reduce the "adjustment period" for a new staff member, increase loyalty, reduce accidents, reduce waste, and eliminate violation of important rules due to ignorance.

COMPARISON OF CANDIDATES TO POSITION REQUIREMENTS

POSITION TO BE FILLED_____

Rate each candidate using the following scale:				CANDIDATES:		
1. Candidate does not meet this job requirement.						
2. Candidate meets this job requirement.						
3. Candidate exceeds this requirement.						
JOB REQUIREMENTS				**RANKING:**		
General knowledge requirements:						
1.						
2.						
3.						
4.						
5.						
Specific job skills and/or knowledge:						
1.						
2.						
3.						
4.						
5.						
Education or training required:						
1.						
2.						
3.						
4.						
5.						
TOTALS						

General Guidelines

When getting ready to welcome new staff members, remember that they may be tired and bewildered by too much new information and too many new faces. Newcomers do well if they remember a fraction of what they have been told, and appreciate a nurse supervisor who doesn't mind repeating information. Keep the following guidelines in mind when orienting new employees:

Make a good first impression. Greet the new staff member. Smile. Shake hands. Use the person's name—check to see if first names are okay. Be friendly. Make small talk. Ask about the commute. Make it clear that this is a terrific place to work. Let your pride in your unit show. Let new staff members know you are confident in them.

Describe the work. Show the new staff member how the job fits into the health care facility as a whole.

Furnish essential information. Newcomers have already heard more than they can remember. The essential information includes

- patient/client assignment procedures.
- orientation class schedules.
- pay-procedures and schedules.
- parking and transportation.
- breaks, including lunch—where to go and how long to take.
- unit layout—client rooms, utility rooms, staff lockers, equipment, and supplies.
- attendance—procedures for absences, clocking in and out, and work hours.
- phone numbers—where the new staff member can be reached by family members in an emergency.

Introduce the new staff member. Take the opportunity to say a good word about each person you introduce to the new staff member. Not only does it help the newcomer get to know people more quickly, it's also good for everyone's morale. Introduce the "buddy" last. A "buddy" is a staff member who has agreed to work with the new staff member for a specified amount of time, until the new person is comfortable working independently on the unit.

Arrange a lunch date. Make sure you or someone else who is friendly and supportive invites the new person to lunch.

Check back. Don't hang over the shoulder of a new staff member, but do check back during the day and at the end of the day to see how things are going.

If a work emergency prevents you from orienting a new staff member yourself, ask a trusted staff nurse or other subordinate to take over. Introduce your "substitute" to the new staff member and explain why you can't do the honors yourself.

Health Care Facility Orientation

The Department of Human Resources (DHR) provides a formal orientation for new staff. Most health care facility orientation programs offer a brief history of the facility, its organization, regulations and policies, training opportunities, special benefits, retirement, the credit union, and any staff assistance programs. Training programs such as ergonomics, fire safety, and infection control procedures are opportunities that may need to be scheduled prior to a new employee working in your unit. Health care facilities have differing policies, but many require completion of essential programs prior to the employee's first day on the job. Check with your DHR to find out what training has to be completed before you are permitted to schedule new staff members for their first day of work on your unit.

EXAM QUESTIONS

CHAPTER 10
Questions 75–81

75. What one word must characterize the interviewing process in order to uphold Title VII of the Civil Rights Act?

    a. formal

    b. projection

    c. objectivity

    d. open

76. What is one of the questions you must ask yourself when analyzing a vacant position?

    a. What skills and knowledge are necessary to perform the job?

    b. What type of personality does this job take?

    c. Who would best fit this type of job?

    d. How can I follow the agency norm in selecting the right candidate?

77. Which statement best describes the use of lead questions in job interviews?

    a. Different lead questions should be asked of each candidate.

    b. The same lead questions should be asked of each candidate.

    c. Lead questions should be asked at the end of the interview.

    d. Lead questions should be used very carefully, because they can lead to law suits.

78. Questions beginning with _____ are likely to produce the most informative answers.

    a. "have you" and "did you"

    b. "what" and "tell me"

    c. "when did" and "are you"

    d. "how many" and "will you"

79. Which of the following questions is an acceptable interview question?

    a. Are you a U.S. citizen?

    b. When did you go to college?

    c. What type of military discharge did you receive?

    d. Do you belong to any general community organizations?

80. What will the best candidate for any position have besides the best job-related pattern of critical strengths?

    a. least complaints about previous jobs

    b. most years in Civil Service

    c. no conviction records

    d. fewest serious limitations

81. The three essential pieces of information you need to supply to the new staff nurse on the first day are

    a. sick time, holidays, vacation.

    b. patient/client assignment procedures, unit layout, parking.

    c. grievances, pay increases, staffing policy.

    d. evaluation procedures, overtime pay, probation period.

CHAPTER 11

TRAINING NURSING STAFF

INTRODUCTION

In this chapter, you will learn about the supervisor's role in training staff. We will talk about what training is, which work situations create a need for training, how to analyze a job or task so that you can help someone learn to do it, and how to create a training plan. You will have opportunities to practice some training planning skills.

CHAPTER OBJECTIVES

After studying this chapter, you will be able to recognize the nurse supervisor's function in training nursing staff.

LEARNING OBJECTIVES

Upon completion of this chapter, you will be able to:

1. Identify examples of performance problems that represent non-training needs.

2. Recognize the elements of a training plan.

3. Specify verbs that are appropriate for use in a learning objective.

4. Identify the steps taken to analyze a performance discrepancy.

LESSON CONTENT

If you're a nurse supervisor, you are probably already familiar with training. You conduct training when you

• correct staff member's performance or answer a question.

• give direction to a staff member.

• explain regulations or procedures.

• conduct special meetings.

• orient new staff.

A formal training program puts those skills to use in a more structured way.

IS TRAINING THE ANSWER?

Some work situations automatically create a need for training. For example

• changes in laws, programs, or procedures. Changes in "Code Blue" procedures create a need for training for all health care facility staff.

• advances in science and technology. Switching from handwritten nurses' notes to those entered on a computer creates a need for training.

• staff members who want to be promoted. Expanding the tasks a staff member handles creates a need for training.

In addition, nurse supervisors sometimes provide training to correct poor performance and sometimes offer training as a reward to staff who have potential and have performed well.

However, not all performance problems are training problems. Performance problems include

- poor quality client care.

- incomplete nurse's notes.

- failure to complete client care by the end of shift.

- low morale.

- excessive turnover.

- excessive absenteeism.

- large numbers of complaints and grievances.

- confusion or bickering over lines of authority.

- high number of "incident reports."

- nurse supervisors regularly performing routine tasks.

This is a list of symptoms. Their causes could range from poor hiring practices to inefficient management to physical disorganization. "Throwing training" at every performance problem that comes up is both inefficient and ineffective. Nurse supervisors must determine whether training can solve a particular problem.

To make this determination, nurse supervisors can use a five-step procedure explained in the performance narrative that follows. The procedures are illustrated in the flow chart that follows (adapted from Mager, 1997).

PERFORMANCE PROBLEM ANALYSIS FLOW

STEP 1 **Describe the performance discrepancy.** For this step you'll answer the question, What is the difference between what is being done and what is supposed to be done?

STEP 2 **Decide whether the problem is important enough to try to solve.** Some problems are insignificant. Some problems, left alone, solve themselves. To decide whether a problem is worth the effort it would take to correct it, ask yourself, What does this problem cost the health care facility? or Does this problem reduce quality of client care? What are the likely consequences of simply ignoring the problem? If the problem can't be ignored, go on to Step 3.

STEP 3 **Decide whether an important problem is the result of a skill deficiency.** Ask yourself, Could this person (or these people) give the correct performance if his or her life depended on it? If the staff member is capable of the performance but isn't doing it, the solution to your problem lies with some area other than training. Perhaps there is a motivation problem or something that prevents the staff member from performing correctly. Check with your supervisor for help. If the staff member couldn't possibly perform the task, you are dealing with a skill deficiency. You don't necessarily have a training problem, though. Go to Step 4.

STEP 4 **Determine whether the staff member with the skill deficiency used to be able to perform the skill.** Ask yourself, Did the person once know how to perform the task? Has he or she forgotten how? If the answer is No, your staff member needs formal training. If the answer is Yes, go to Step 5.

STEP 5 **Determine frequency of use.** Ask yourself, how often is the skill used? Is there regular feedback on quality of performance? Exactly how does the person find out how well he or she is doing? People tend to forget skills when they use them infrequently, unless they practice them. Skills used often but without any feedback on quality can become sloppy. In either case, you won't need formal training to solve this problem—just practice or feedback, as the case may be.

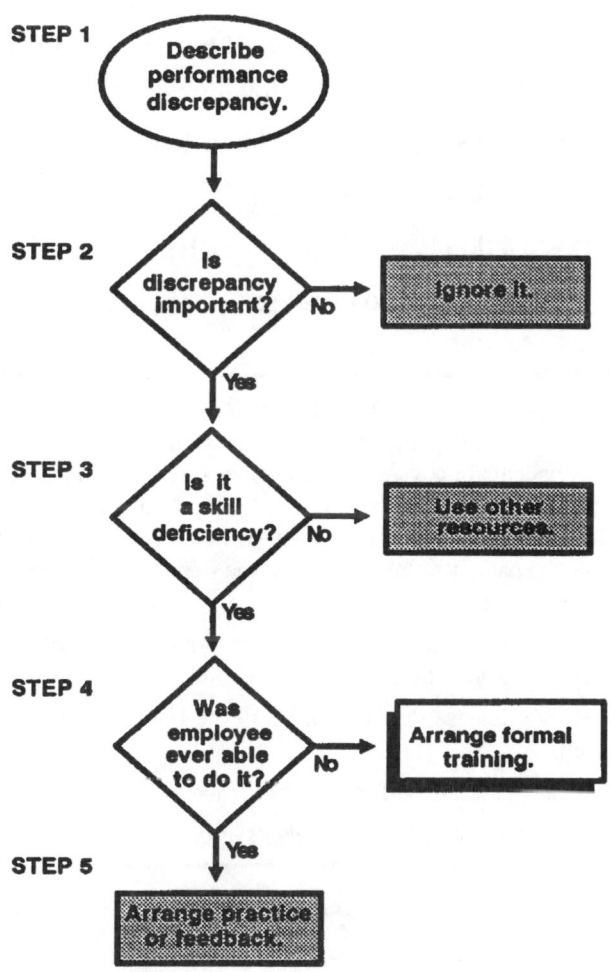

PERFORMANCE PROBLEM ANALYSIS FLOW CHART
(adapted from Mager, 1997)

ACTIVITY

Even the best health care facility units have some function that could be improved. Select a performance problem within your unit. (Are Intake and Output sheets being completed? Are nurses'

notes left incomplete? Is routine clean-up after shifts being ignored?) Analyze it according to the Performance Problem Analysis Flow Chart.

> ### Example
> Sherry Jackson is a unit manager who was a great advocate of training. Sherry's supervisor helped her distinguish whether a performance problem is also a training problem:
> 1. Sherry's fellow worker yelled at clients three times one week. Sherry advocated a course in Stress Management, Dealing with Anger, or Communication Skills. After meeting with the person and discussing the situation, Sherry's supervisor made a referral to the medical facility's Employee Assistance Program. The co-worker had handled clients well for the preceding year, so obviously had the skills to deal with stress and anger.
> 2. Clients had lodged seven complaints against another of Sherry's fellow workers. Sherry advocated Stress Management, Dealing with Anger, or Communication Skills. Sherry's supervisor sat in with the staff member for the next few interviews and practiced some role-playing with her later. The staff member was sent to a course called "Dealing with Difficult People" the next week. Sherry's supervisor and the staff member had agreed on goals with learning before selecting the course. In follow-up sessions, Sherry's supervisor and the staff member reviewed and discussed the extent to which the learning goals had been met. They again role-played, with much better results.

TRAINING RESOURCES

Once you've determined that you have a genuine training problem, you need to figure out how to provide the training needed. You won't necessarily have to do the training yourself. You can

• arrange for training with another unit.

• arrange for training with your Health Care Facility Safety Officer or Director of Training.

• refer staff to outside programs.

• enlist the aid of other staff as trainers.

• refer staff to self-guided or home-study courses.

ON-THE-JOB TRAINING

Sometimes the best way to address a training need is to teach the needed skills during the work day, at the work site. This type of training is called on-the-job training (OJT).

OJT is learning by doing the job. While most nurses, even as new graduates come out of nursing school with basic clinical skills, many nurses will be in need of reviews on how to perform these skills with your health care facility's supplies and equipment. Additionally, many procedures, for example working with a kidney dialysis machine or working as a scrub nurse in O.R., take special training. This need exists because the practice of nursing is so diverse, it is not possible for nurses to be accomplished in all the specialty areas that exist. This training is either done OJT or in special courses developed by the health care facility.

A systematic approach to OJT—like the one described below—will help you get new staff into production faster and will allow you to quickly train old hands in new procedures.

Pros and Cons of On-the-Job Training

OJT has several advantages over other training methods. These advantages include

- learners can improve their skills under real-world conditions.

- training can be made specific to the job and to the individual.

- training can be carried out on a one-to-one basis.

- it saves time that other methods use up in traveling to a specific training location.

- it costs nothing in course fees or tuition.

Its disadvantages include

- it costs staff trainer time.

- it often interferes with efficient client care.

- workplace distractions can interfere with training.

- not all staff trainers are efficient, organized instructors.

Preparing an OJT Lesson

An effective OJT unit can be prepared in four short steps.

STEP 1 Analyze the job.

In this step, you tell yourself how a job should be done. Ask yourself the following questions:

- "What steps do I go through to do this job?"

- "What happens at each step?"

- "What do I have to know at each step?"

- "In what order do the steps take place?"

Example

In the emergency room, nurses are frequently faced with patients in advanced stages of shock. It is difficult to auscultate the blood pressure in these patients without a Doppler. A nurse working in the ER is expected to estimate the patient's blood pressure. The steps that need to be performed are:

- Record the mmHg corresponding to the first pulsation they palpate as the systolic B/P.
- Slowly release the B/P cuff until the brachial pulse is felt.
- Inflating the B/P cuff until the brachial pulse is obliterated.
- Place the B/P cuff on the patient's arm.

ACTIVITY

Using a separate sheet of paper, arrange the steps in the example above in correct order. When you're finished, check your work against the list that follows.

In this example, the tasks are all there, but they need to be arranged in logical sequence. The logical sequence would be as follows:

1. Place the B/P cuff on the patient's arm.

2. Inflate the B/P cuff until the brachial pulse is obliterated.

3. Slowly release the B/P cuff until the brachial pulse is felt.

4. Record the mmHg corresponding to the first pulsation as the systolic B/P.

Now expand your list. Under each task list all the things a nurse must know or be able to do to accomplish that task. Try to remember what it was like to be new at the job. Don't make any assumptions about what the person will know. For instance, don't assume the person remembers where to palpate the brachial artery. Write it on your list.

STEP 2 Set training objectives.

An objective is a statement of **what** the learner will be able to do when the training is completed. It also specifies **how well** the learner will be able to do it. It gives the learner a target to shoot for. It defines success. It provides the basis for evaluation of the completed training. It also can inform the person of the standard for the job.

Objectives are based on **observable behavior,** so both the trainer and the trainee will know when the task has been learned. The key to developing good, observable training objectives is **active verbs:** *pump, write, drive, lift.* You could watch someone pump, write or lift. Try observing someone *appreciate, understand, internalize,* or *feel.*

Example

OBSERVABLE: Given a sterile dressing kit, change a dressing using sterile technique.

NOT OBSERVABLE: Be able to demonstrate an understanding of the principles of sterile technique for changing dressings.

OBSERVABLE: Perform the steps in starting an intravenous fluid drip.

NOT OBSERVABLE: Understand the procedure for starting an intravenous drip.

One training expert offers the "Hey, Dad" test to determine whether an objective is observable. To do this, he says, you use the substance of your objective to finish this sentence: "Hey, Dad, let me show you how I can _____." You can't show someone how you can appreciate art. However, you can show someone how you can type a letter.

The part of an objective that states how well the learner should perform the task is the standard. Standards include limiting factors such as time, numbers, and percentages.

Example

TIME: Make six home visits in a day.

NUMBER: Estimate the systolic B/P of five patients.

PERCENTAGE: Estimate all systolic B/Ps with 100% accuracy.

ACTIVITY

Select a simple task—placing a telephone call to order supplies, filling out a laboratory request, taking a patient's temperature—and analyze it on a separate piece of paper. Then write objectives for each of the subtasks that make up the task.

Evaluate your work by checking it against the following criteria:

1. Does each objective make sense when put to the "Hey, Dad" test ("Hey, Dad, let me show you how I can _____.")?

2. Does each objective contain a standard (how fast, how many, in what manner, etc.)?

If you can answer yes to each question, you've written usable objectives. You're ready for Step 3. If your answer to either question was no, rework your objectives.

STEP 3 Schedule Facilities.

Make sure all arrangements for OJT have been made well before the actual session begins. Consider the following:

Time. Estimate and schedule time for the session without interruptions.

Space. Make sure there is enough space available, it has been scheduled for OJT, and it is big enough for OJT.

Training aids. Make sure tools, equipment, and supplies are available and are working.

Client/Patient Care. Make sure OJT will not interrupt regular client care demands. If the client census is unusually high, you may need to reschedule.

STEP 4 **Create an Instruction Plan.**

The purpose of the instruction plan is to organize the work you've already done into chart form so that you can refer to it during the session. Keep in mind that people usually can remember about seven points in a single lesson.

ACTIVITY

Following the example, make an instruction plan for the task you analyzed earlier in this section. Compare your plan with the example above for completeness.

CONDUCTING OJT

Now you're ready to conduct OJT. An OJT session consists of five steps.

OJT INSTRUCTION PLAN

OBJECTIVES: At the end of the session, the learner will be able to _____

_____

_____

TRAINING AIDS: (Tools, equipment, forms, etc.) _____

_____

_____

TRAINING METHODS: _____

_____

_____

STEP #	TASK	PROCEDURE	REASON

STEP 1 Prepare the learner.

STEP 2 Demonstrate the job.

STEP 3 Watch while learner practices the job.

STEP 4 Allow the learner to work alone.

STEP 5 Give the learner feedback. Repeat Steps 3 and 4 if necessary.

This system is similar to others you might have heard of. Sometimes the steps are referred to as "You say, you do; you say, they do; they say, they do."

TRAINING RECORDS

Up-to-date training records are crucial to a staff member's career. Promotions, demotions, and performance appraisals often refer to the contents of a staff member's training file. Some health care facilities require units to keep their own training records. If you are going to keep your staff members' records, you'll use them to note what they've done and what they're going to do, both in OJT and other training.

Training records should show a step-by-step training program for each staff member. Each step should be signed and dated by the person responsible for the training when the staff member finishes it. Records should also contain a rough schedule for upcoming training.

Training records can be used in performance appraisals.

Your health care facility may have an automated system for tracking staff member's training, including information on available courses and records of what each staff member has completed and still needs. Check with the nursing department's training coordinator.

STEP 1. Prepare the learner.

PURPOSE	METHODS
Put the learner at ease.	Keep a friendly attitude. Speak slowly. Tell learner she or he will have plenty of time to learn. Express confidence in learner's ability.
Tie in today's lesson with learner's knowledge and background.	Find out learner's background. Show relation of learner's existing skills to new task.
Secure the learner's attention, arouse his or her interest, and create a desire to learn.	Be enthusiastic. State the job to be learned. Explain job's importance and significance. Give the learner the "big picture"—how this task ties in to the function of the unit. Tell learner the advantages of learning this job.

STEP 2. Demonstrate the job.

PURPOSE	METHODS
Show and explain the job.	Use your OJT Instruction Plan.
	Go SLOWLY—gauge speed to learner.
	Identify key points and sequence.
	Emphasize safety.
	Define any specialized nursing or medical terms.

	Demonstrate task:
	    If working with machinery, place learner in same position and facing the same direction as yourself.
	    Perform the entire task yourself. Stress safety.
	    Repeat the demonstration step by step, explaining each step and why and how it is done.
	    Check for questions.

	Give related information.
	MOST PEOPLE REMEMBER ABOUT SEVEN POINTS IN A SINGLE LESSON!

STEP 3. Watch while learner practices the job.

PURPOSE	METHODS
Let the learner do the job under supervision.	Change places with learner. Allow him or her to do the job, explaining what he or she is going to do **before** each step. Summarize key points.
Help the learner develop confidence.	Praise him or her. Be specific. Let him or her do the job several times under supervision.
Correct learner's errors.	Watch carefully. Correct learner before he or she makes an error. Reteach if necessary. Be patient.
Verify that learner understands.	Ask open-ended questions about each step. Let learner go through job without interruption.
Help the learner develop good work habits.	Stress key points. Emphasize correct practice and safety. Show "tricks of the trade" to make work easy.
Reteach if necessary.	Repeat demonstration.

STEP 4. Allow learner to work alone.

PURPOSE	METHODS
See if learner can work independently.	Put learner on his or her own. Tell him or her where to go for help.
Show continued interest in learner's work and growth.	Check back occasionally. Give additional information and shortcuts. Encourage questions and suggestions. Avoid fault-finding. Give specific praise.

STEP 5. Give the learner feedback. Repeat Steps 3 and 4 if necessary.

PURPOSE	METHODS
Determine the extent of learning, skills that require reteaching, and effectiveness of instruction.	Observe and verify performance.

SUPPLEMENTAL ACTIVITY

1. Meet with your boss or nurse supervisor and discuss the methods he or she uses to organize OJT. Discuss some of the performance prob-lems you have seen on the unit. After validating that the performance problem represents a need for training, use the following OJT Instruction Plan to plan instruction to correct the problem.

EMPLOYEE: Gilborn, Jane L.				
OJT TRAINING SCHEDULE				
JOB	PROJECTED TRAINING DATE	ACTUAL TRAINING DATE	TRAINER	VERIFIED COMPLETED
Calculate Lidocaine Drip	4/3/96	4/3/96	Clark, A.J.	LPQ
Operation of IABP	4/15/96	4/2/96	Quince, L.P.	LPQ
Estimate B/P without Doppler	5/10/96			
Operation of Hypothermia Machine	6/1/96			
GENERAL TRAINING SCHEDULE				
Orientation	3/25/96	3/25/96	Training	LPQ

OJT INSTRUCTION PLAN

OBJECTIVES: At the end of the session, the learner will be able to _____

_____

_____

TRAINING AIDS: (Tools, equipment, forms, etc.) _____

_____

_____

TRAINING METHODS: _____

_____

_____

STEP #	TASK	PROCEDURE	REASON

EXAM QUESTIONS

CHAPTER 11
Questions 82–86

82. What is indicated by failures to complete client care, incomplete nurses' notes, and excessive turnover?

    a. poor leadership

    b. a need for training

    c. performance problems

    d. poor hiring practices

83. If a performance discrepancy is a skill deficiency that a staff member once had but has lost, what should the nurse supervisor do?

    a. ignore it

    b. arrange formal training

    c. use other resources

    d. arrange practice and feedback

84. You've completed the job analysis and developed the training objectives. What's next?

    a. develop the final product

    b. schedule facilities

    c. create the instruction plan

    d. develop the course goals

85. You are preparing a unit of OJT for the nurses in an ICU. You ask yourself, what are the steps that one must take to do a job? Exactly what happens at each step? What is the prerequisite knowledge to perform each step?

    What step of training development are you performing?

    a. developing objectives

    b. setting goals

    c. developing remediation

    d. analyzing the job

86. Which of the following verbs is observable and appropriate for use in a learning objective?

    a. understand

    b. synthesize

    c. appreciate

    d. perform

CHAPTER 12

PERFORMANCE APPRAISALS

INTRODUCTION

In this chapter, we'll talk about the place of performance appraisals in nursing and in the careers of nurse supervisors and the people they supervise. You'll learn how to prepare for an appraisal, how to prepare a performance report, and what to cover in a performance report discussion with a staff member. We'll also discuss ways to help improve staff performance and ways to help staff "keep up the good work."

CHAPTER OBJECTIVE

After studying this chapter, you will be able to identify appropriate methods for conducting performance appraisals.

LEARNING OBJECTIVES

Upon completion of this chapter, you will be able to:

1. Recognize the benefits of regular performance appraisals for the health care facility and the staff member.

2. Specify the steps involved in preparing for a performance appraisal.

3. Identify the steps involved in discussing a performance report with a staff member.

4. Recognize guidelines for dealing with the need for improved performance.

5. State techniques for recognizing good performance and maintaining improved performance.

LESSON CONTENT

One of the most challenging and rewarding functions of nurses who supervise others is that of appraising performance. It is in this capacity that supervisors are able to help the staff they supervise improve professionally.

Valuable staff members grow constantly in their jobs. As nurse supervisor, you play a critical role in stimulating that growth. Performance appraisals are one way to help staff improve—whether their current performance is adequate, inadequate, or outstanding.

PERFORMANCE APPRAISAL IS A PROCESS

Although an "official" appraisal may happen only a few times a year, the process of appraising performance goes on all the time. As a nurse supervisor, you are responsible for helping your staff develop professionally. That means you must keep current on opportuni programs, and procedures that can help nursing department and health c that arrive in your in-basket and are posted on bulletin boards. Get to know your director of training and/or people in the Human Resources Department. As you receive information on new training programs and promotional opportunities, pass it on to your staff.

Be able to explain health care facility procedures to your staff. Never assume that staff members understand the selection process, transfer policies, tuition reimbursement programs, or other opportunities.

Document typical and significant examples of both good and poor performance. Meet with staff regularly to advise them of their progress, not just when the health care facility regulations require you to do so. In general, staff should have access to all information about them recorded by their nurse supervisor. Check with the Human Resources Department if you have a question about this policy.

You can't expect miracles from this process. However, you can expect to see your staff grow and improve if you base your development plans on solid foundations of trust and communication. And don't be surprised if you find that you receive even more from the process than your staff member.

Why Rate Staff Performance?

Performance appraisals require a real time commitment on the part of the nurse supervisor. They become valuable tools for both staff and supervisors when used correctly. Used incorrectly, they can become superficial or destructive and can lead to bad feelings between the supervisor and the staff member. Additionally, many nurse supervisors feel very uncomfortable about appraising the performance of staff members who were recently their co-workers. With all this in mind, why do you think it is important to rate staff performance?

ACTIVITY

List as many reasons as you can think of for rating staff performance: _____

_____

_____

_____

_____

_____

_____

Performance appraisals fulfill a number of needs for both the staff and the health care facility. Your list could contain at least a few of the following items. Appraisals help staff to:

- Perform their jobs more easily and effectively.

- Prepare for advancement.

- Improve future performance.

- Clarify new responsibilities that have evolved in their jobs.

Appraisals help the health care facility and the nurse supervisor to:

- Provide frank and constructive feedback to the staff member.

- Recognize past performance.

- Assist staff in performing their jobs more easily and effectively.

- Maintain standards of performance.

- Stay aware of how effectively and economically work is being performed.

- Relate compensation to performance.

- Make decisions in transfers, suspensions, demotions, and removals.

Most staff members say appraisals allow them to know "where they stand" with their supervisors, which helps lower their anxiety. Lower anxiety usually means higher productivity—a benefit for staff, clients, and the health care facility. Staff members want help in goal setting and coaching on ways to improve future performance (Sullivan, 1994). Furthermore, appraisals provide insight for nurse supervisors into how the job is evolving and how those who perform the job prioritize job tasks.

Unfortunately some organizations have staff evaluation procedures that are inconsistent, subjective, and even unknown to the staff members. Fair and objective staff evaluation procedures should include

- Standards that are clear, objective, and known in advance.

- Uniformly applied criteria for pay raises and promotions.

- Known conditions under which employment may be terminated.

- Open access for staff to inspect their personnel files.

- A reasonable amount of time for staff to correct serious deficiencies before action is taken.

- Opportunity for the staff to appeal a rating if they do not agree with it.

HOW OFTEN?

There are a number of occasions for appraisals. In most health care facilities, staff performance reports are scheduled for mid-probation and final probation. Most health care facilities consider the probationary period to be an extension of the selection process. Periodic appraisals during the probationary period allow the staff member and nurse supervisor to stay up-to-date on the staff member's performance. Each health care facility has set periodic performance appraisals (usually every six months to one year) after the probationary period.

Other occasions for appraisals are promotion, transfer, demotion, and separation. Performance reports are also used when there is a need for special documentation of performance. They can be used to report outstanding performance or below standard performance during the rating period. Nurse supervisors leaving their work units, for instance, should fill out performance reports for their successors' reference, even if it has been less than a year since the last report for some staff members.

PERFORMANCE STANDARDS

Appraisal and development should be measured against established standards. Using written standards makes appraisal easier and fairer. For appraisals to be effective, each staff member must know and understand the standards.

The Standards of Nursing Practice of the American Nurses Association is a good source for developing standards for the practice of nursing. In many organizations, job descriptions also are used as an evaluation tool for performance appraisals. Job descriptions should spell out the essential job functions and should include responsibilities, activities to be performed, and any results expected of the staff member. The time to explain the job descriptions and standards to staff is when they first begin working for you—make it part of your orientation program.

There should be NO SURPRISES for a staff member during a performance appraisal. A staff member who the nurse supervisor thinks is doing the job at or above the standard should know that's what the nurse supervisor thinks. Whether the person's performance ratings are unsatisfactory, standard, or above standard, they should be kept informed at regular intervals by their nurse supervisor.

PREPARING FOR THE REVIEW

Before reviews, remind staff to prepare. Offer the list of questions—Employee Self-Appraisal: Food for Thought—as a guide.

For your own preparation, pull the staff member's written records. These could include departmental records for the current appraisal period (and possibly old appraisals), as well as your own records. (Of course, your own records must not be "secret." If you keep notes on a staff member's performance—positive or negative—you should make those notes available for the staff member's inspection. If you have questions about what to record and how to describe it, check with your supervisor or personnel department.) Use a form like the one in chapter 12, called "Nurse Supervisor's Review Notes for Performance Appraisal," to review the records.

Do not plan the content of the interview too firmly; you may want to alter your approach to what appears to concern the staff member.

Provide a **private meeting place.** Allow plenty of time. Arrange not to be interrupted.

EMPLOYEE SELF-APPRAISAL: FOOD FOR THOUGHT

THE PAST AND THE PRESENT   Date _____

1. What critical abilities does my job require? To what extent do I fulfill them? _____

   _____

2. What do I like best about my job? Least? _____

   _____

3. What were my specific accomplishments during this appraisal period? _____

   _____

4. Which goals or standards did I fall short of meeting? _____

   _____

5. What have I done since my last appraisal to prepare myself for more responsibility? _____

   _____

6. Does my present job make the best use of my capabilities? How could I become more productive? _____

   _____

MY NURSE SUPERVISOR'S PERFORMANCE

7. How could my nurse supervisor help me do a better job? _____

   _____

8. Is there anything that the organization or my nurse supervisor does that hinders my effectiveness? _____

   _____

9. What changes would improve my performance? _____

   _____

THE FUTURE

10. What do I expect to be doing five years from now? _____

   _____

11. Do I need more experience or training in any aspect of my current job? How could it be accomplished?

   _____

12. What new goals and standards should be established for the next appraisal period? Which old ones need

to be modified or deleted? _____

NURSE SUPERVISOR'S REVIEW NOTES FOR PERFORMANCE APPRAISAL

STAFF MEMBER:_____ DATE _____

THE PAST AND THE PRESENT

1. What are this staff member's past objectives, achievements, and performance? _____
    _____

2. What critical abilities does this job require? To what extent does this staff member fulfill them? _____
    _____

3. What was covered in previous talks? What has this staff member accomplished since then? _____
    _____

4. What standards does this staff member fall short of meeting? _____
    _____

MY PERFORMANCE IN SUPERVISING THIS STAFF MEMBER

5. What have I done to assist this staff member to do a good job? _____
    _____

6. What have I done that may have hindered this staff member in doing his or her job? _____
    _____

THE FUTURE

7. What is this staff member likely to want to know about salary, opportunities, policies, performance?_____
    _____

8. What new goals and standards should be established for the next appraisal period? _____
    _____

9. Which old goals and standards should be deleted? _____
    _____

PREPARING THE PERFORMANCE REPORT

Before preparing a performance report, check with your personnel department. You may need to fill out different performance report forms for the people you supervise in different departments. For example, your nursing staff are considered a part of the nursing department, while your ward secretaries may be considered part of the facility's clerical department. These guidelines will give you a general idea of how to complete a performance report.

1. Consult with other supervisors that the staff member had during the rating period.

2. Mark the report in pencil.

   • Base all ratings on **facts.** You should be able to document and explain all ratings other than what is standard.

   • Resist any temptation to

      — rate a staff member high on everything because of a few strong points or low on everything because of a few weaknesses.

      — rate all staff high or all staff low.

      — play it safe by automatically rating all staff as standard.

   • Be consistent. Rate staff members who perform the same level and type of work by the same standards.

   • Use the comment section for ratings that require explanation. Include staff member performance you have actually observed. Describe consequences of the staff member's performance.

   • Evaluate **only job-related behaviors.** Be aware of your own values; do not reward or penalize staff members for their values or for their personalities.

   • Include comments on the staff member's

demonstrated potential for promotion, improvement to date, performance objectives, and other matters related to continuing professional development.

3. Review the report with your supervisor.

STRUCTURING THE PERFORMANCE REPORT DISCUSSION

There are various customs for carrying out the report discussion. In some health care facilities, nurse supervisors meet with staff to discuss the performance report. If you as a nurse supervisor are to meet with staff you've rated, you'll need to prepare for the meeting. Remember, your first priority is to find a private space and a block of uninterrupted time.

Your general appraisal—anywhere from "unsatisfactory" to "superior"—will determine the course of your discussion with a staff member.

If your general appraisal is **superior,** your discussion should center on:
   • Ways to maintain current performance level.
   • Possibility of extending responsibility.
   • Development plans.
   • Opportunities for advancement.

If your general appraisal is **satisfactory,** your discussion should center on:
   • Ways to maintain or improve the performance level.
   • Development plans.
   • Possibilities for advancement.

If your general appraisal is **unsatisfactory,** your discussion should center on:
   • Where performance is deficient.
   • Plans for correction.
   • Gaining a commitment for correction.
   • Possibility of reassignment or termination.

ACTIVITY

Think about your own last performance report discussion. Describe how you felt. Why did you feel that way? What happened to help you feel good about your job? How might things have been done differently?

Activity Feedback

Hopefully you felt good about your last performance report discussion. The reasons might be

- there were no surprises. You already knew your supervisor thought you were doing an outstanding job.

- you already knew what concerns your supervisor had and you had been thinking of ways to solve the problem.

- you were pleased to have this special one-on-one time with your supervisor.

- you are pleased with the opportunity to work on the project the supervisor suggested.

COMMUNICATION SKILLS FOR THE PERFORMANCE REPORT DISCUSSION

Many of the guidelines for conducting an interview apply to your appraisal report discussion. You should

- Conduct the interview in private—no interruptions.

- Keep your tone friendly.

- Be aware of your personal biases, and keep them out of the discussion.

- Avoid arguing and cross-examining.

Before your appointment, review the concepts of good communication presented earlier in this course. Especially keep in mind the material on lis-

tening skills. A successful discussion is one in which the staff member does most of the talking. To convince a staff member to talk freely with you:

- **Be descriptive rather than judgmental.** Being judgmental will almost certainly make your staff member feel defensive. Describing behavior in objective terms allows an objective discussion.

  JUDGMENTAL: "How could you do such a dumb thing?"

  DESCRIPTIVE: "Can you explain what caused the incident?"

- **Be supportive, not authoritarian.** It can be easy to slip into an authoritarian role—telling a staff member what to do. Being supportive of a staff member's ability to contribute to the solution to a problem creates an atmosphere of mutual respect.

  AUTHORITARIAN: "Here is what we will do to get this done on time."

  SUPPORTIVE: "What do you suggest we do to get this done on time in the future?"

- **Reflect equality, not superiority.** You create a barrier to communication when you put too much emphasis on the power that comes with your position as the staff member's nurse supervisor. Ask for opinions and listen to ideas. If you do, you're likely to find that staff talk openly with you, rather than "tune you out."

  REFLECTS SUPERIORITY: "I was doing it this way before you were born."

  REFLECTS EQUALITY: "We have done it this way for years, but I would like to hear your ideas on how we can do it better."

- **Be accepting, not dogmatic.** When you accept staff member input, you capitalize on knowledge, build confidence in the group, and stimulate enthusiasm and creativity. What happens in your private discussions with staff becomes part of your reputation as a nurse supervisor-not necessarily the content, but the attitude you convey.

DOGMATIC: "This is the best solution."

ACCEPTING: "This is the best solution I could come up with. What other possibilities do you see?"

ACTIVITY

Rewrite the following statements to make them:

- Descriptive rather than judgmental.

- Supportive rather than authoritarian.

- Reflective of equality, not superiority.

- Accepting, not dogmatic.

1. Did you really think that plan would work?

Rewrite: _____

_____

_____

2. We tried it that way five years ago. It didn't work then, and it won't work now.

Rewrite: _____

_____

_____

3. I would expect even a new person to have better sense than that.

Rewrite: _____

_____

_____

Activity Feedback

If you noticed that item #1 is judgmental, congratulations! You might say something like, "What do you think went wrong?"

Item #2 reflects the superior "I've already been there" attitude. Perhaps use a statement like, "Let's look together at what has changed since we tried this approach five years ago. Maybe the situation is different enough now to do it successfully."

Item #3 is judgmental. Help the staff member see the consequences of a problem: "What was the result of that? How could it be changed to achieve the result we want?"

CONDUCTING THE PERFORMANCE REPORT DISCUSSION

With these pointers firmly in mind, you're ready to begin the discussion. The following steps will help you stay on track. (Check with your supervisor first; not all departments follow the general guidelines described below.)

STEP 1 **Start with a positive achievement.** Some nurse supervisors start by asking staff to sum up their achievements for the review period. Others ask how they can help make the job easier or more effectively done.

STEP 2 **Discuss needed improvements.** Describe the impact of any unsatisfactory performance on the work unit. Make sure the staff member is aware of the performance standards for any tasks for which performance is rated below "standard."

STEP 3 **Ask for ideas for making improvements or development.** Together, work out a plan for improvement or development. High-achieving staff members need a plan, too, for their development. This may include training, self-instruction, etc. Use your best objective-writing skills. Make sure the staff member's plan includes objectives that are measurable, challenging, and attainable. Ask the staff member to commit to achieving the goals within a reasonable amount of time, and set a date for the next review to check progress, which can be before the next formal appraisal.

STEP 4 **Give the staff member an opportunity to discuss ratings.** Use your best listening skills here. Your supervisor can tell you about your departmental policy: some departments have the final report typed, some have the nurse supervisor fill it out in ink. Request the staff member to sign the form to indicate that the ratings have been discussed. Make it clear that the staff member's signature indicates that the staff member has reviewed the appraisal and may or may not agree with it. Give the staff member a copy after all signatures have been made.

Explain the Appeal Process

It should be clear to staff that they can appeal a performance report. Plan to go over the report again with your supervisor if the staff member makes a protest. If they refuse to sign to acknowledge that they have seen and discussed it, note this on the appraisal form and then route it through normal channels. If a prior appraisal was below standard, a staff member should receive, if requested, a supplemental appraisal midway through the staff member's next appraisal cycle.

THE UNSATISFACTORY PERFORMANCE REPORT DISCUSSION

Conducting a performance appraisal for a highly motivated staff member is usually a satisfying experience for both the staff member and the nurse supervisor. However, conducting a performance appraisal for a staff member who has unsatisfactory performance can be very uncomfortable. Many nurse supervisors find themselves procrastinating the confrontation of unsatis-

factory performance. Supervisors may rationalize this procrastination by telling themselves

- the behavior is only temporary.

- they want to give the staff member a fair chance.

- the staff member is really a nice person.

- negative feedback will only discourage the staff member.

- the staff member will be leaving or retiring soon.

The failure to confront unsatisfactory behavior is likely to lead to the problem growing, not going away. Other staff members will not ignore the fact that you are letting standards be lowered by tolerating the poor performance. They will become resentful that the person with lower performance is "getting away" with poor performance and is being paid as if their performance were satisfactory. Resentment and lowered morale may ensue from other staff members doing the work the "poor performer" is neglecting. Ultimately, the nurse supervisor who tolerates poor performance is not thought of as a "nice person," but is thought of as ineffective, uncaring, cowardly, and lazy.

Factors Leading to Poor Performance

Unsatisfactory performance may not be the fault of the staff member. There are many reasons for poor performance. One reason stems from the fact that the staff member may have been hired for a job for which *he or she did not have adequate prior experience or education.* For example, the health care facility may have hired the staff member when they were in desperate need of help, and few people were willing to work night shift. The supervisor who hired the staff member might have "made do" with the applicants they had. Other reasons for poor performance include:

- Vague or unrealistic expectations by the health care facility (Tappen, 1995).

- Lack of communication regarding job priorities.

- Poorly developed time management skills.

- Procrastination.

- Lack of confidence.

- Failure to take the initiative.

Resolving the Poor Performance

The first step in resolving a performance problem is to objectively observe and document the problem. Is it a training problem? Does the staff member know how to do it? Review chapter 11 to help you decide.

Once you have documented the performance problem, it is time to have counseling sessions with the staff member. It is tempting for supervisors to wait until the next performance review cycle before they confront performance problems. However, if it is affecting quality of client care or morale, the problem needs immediate attention. It is the nurse supervisor's job to bring problems to the attention of offending staff members and allow them to begin to correct problems as soon as possible. This is best for the offending staff members, and it is fair for the unit as a whole.

The purpose of the session is to communicate the problem and develop a plan for the resolution of the problem. This counseling session may become the first step in disciplinary actions that must follow, if the staff members do not correct poor performance. (Discipline is covered in chapter 13.) Some general guidelines for the counseling session are:

- Calmly identify problems and explain their impact on the unit.

- Encourage staff members to give their reasons for the performance problems.

- Ask staff members if they have ideas for solving the problems.

- Offer to help staff members. (Do they need training? Are they having personal problems? Are they discouraged with, or disinterested in, their present job?)

- Agree on action plans and set a date to review progress concerning problems.

- Focus on the problems, **not the people.**

- Maintain the self-esteem of the staff members.

- Maintain a constructive relationship with the staff members.

MAINTAINING IMPROVED PERFORMANCE

In the best cases—and actually, in most cases-staff will take constructive criticism "to heart" and improve their performance. You may have to meet with a staff member a few more times before any improvement is noted.

Do not ignore improvements—no matter how small!

Praise and reward are two of the most powerful tools you have. Be generous with them. Praise can make a big difference for a staff member who is trying hard to improve. Its absence can demoralize the same staff member.

Incidentally, you don't need to wait for a formal performance appraisal to praise a staff member for improved performance. Anytime you notice a change for the better, comment on it. If improvement has been an issue, schedule a follow-up chat after the performance report discussion, and don't be tempted to cancel it when the staff member "shapes up."

The agenda for a Maintaining Improved Performance discussion is nearly identical to the one you'll use in a Performance Appraisal discussion.

STEP 1   **Describe the improved performance.** Explain the importance of the improvement and the individual's contribution to the unit and the health care facility.

STEP 2 **Give the staff member an opportunity to respond, and listen.**

STEP 3 **Ask if there is anything you can do to make it easier for the staff member to do the job.** When appropriate, make a commitment to take such action.

STEP 4 **Thank the staff member for the improved performance.**

Note: Sometimes performance will improve or staff members will do something "extra" without your having talked to them. Recognize their improvement also.

ACTIVITY

You've noticed that Rachel has taken the initiative to clean out the storage room. This makes it easier for the rest of the staff to find things. Otherwise, Rachel's performance is standard.

What would you say to Rachel?

Activity Feedback

Your comments should be specific. For example

Rachel, thanks for rearranging the storage room. It's so much easier for us to find things. I had been meaning to do it myself. I appreciate your initiative in taking on that project.

SUPPLEMENTAL ACTIVITIES

1. Enlist a co-worker to help you with role-playing. In the scenario, Angie is a staff member who works on the day shift on a medical unit. Things get very busy on the unit, and you are sometimes short-staffed. You have had two complaints from clients and five complaints from other nurses that Angie frequently skips morning baths. She usually says something to the clients or other staff members like, "the P.M. shift can do it, they aren't as busy as we are." Although there are times this is true, she is the only staff member who chronically omits giving her clients baths.

   Have your co-worker pretend she is Angie. Have her complete the *Employee Self-Appraisal: Food for Thought* form. You fill out the *Nurse Supervisor's Review Notes for Performance Appraisal* form. Now conduct a performance appraisal with your co-worker role-playing Angie and you role-playing Angie's supervisor. Use the guidelines in chapter 12 to help you conduct the Performance Appraisal.

EXAM QUESTIONS

CHAPTER 12
Questions 87–95

87. What should staff members do prior to performance appraisals?

    a. write notes about the pitfalls of the current position

    b. review their job descriptions thoroughly

    c. complete staff self-appraisals

    d. write down all of their grievances

88. How do staff performance appraisals help the medical facility?

    a. They help the health care facility provide frank and constructive feedback.

    b. They help determine whether the supervisor is training staff nurses adequately.

    c. They show where the most productive workers are.

    d. They provide insight as to what departments should be closed down.

89. How do performance appraisals help staff nurses?

    a. They let staff nurses know how their supervisors feel about them.

    b. They increase staff nurses' awareness of their chances for demotion.

    c. They provide assurance that they do not need to work hard.

    d. They lower staff nurses' anxiety and increase productivity.

90. Nurse supervisors help staff prepare for Performance Reviews by providing them with

    a. new job descriptions.

    b. employee self-appraisals tools.

    c. past reviews they have received.

    d. documentation of past errors.

91. When conducting a performance report discussion, what should you do first?

    a. identify satisfactory performance

    b. ask for ideas for improvement

    c. identify areas needing improvement

    d. inform the staff member they can appeal the rating

Questions 92–95 address how Mary Wood should conduct Jill Stewart's performance appraisal discussion. Mary supervises Jill. Over the past six months, Jill has had a very poor attendance record. She rarely finishes her client care, frequently asks for special privileges and favors, is uncooperative in group efforts, and is short tempered with co-workers. Overall her job performance appraisal is unsatisfactory.

92. On what should the discussion center?

    a. Jill's opportunities for advancement.

    b. where performance is deficient

    c. the possibility of promotion out of the department

    d. counseling centers Jill can attend

93. Which of the following statements or questions would be most appropriate for Mary to start with?

    a. "Jill, your overall performance is poor, what do you have to say for yourself?"

    b. "Jill, three of your co-workers have complained about your lack of cooperation in helping with tasks that take more than one nurse."

    c. "Jill, do you disagree with any of your ratings?"

    d. "Jill, tell me about your achievements here on the unit in the past six months."

94. Mary discusses the impact of Jill's unsatisfactory performance. What should Mary do next?

    a. Have Jill sign the report.

    b. Talk about the improvements Jill has made.

    c. Ask Jill to help formulate a plan for improvement.

    d. Refer Jill to a higher authority.

95. After two weeks, Mary notes improvement in Jill's cooperative effort. Also, Jill has completed all her client care by the end of her shift. What should Mary do?

    a. Make herself a note to write a report noting the improvements if they continue one month.

    b. Schedule a Maintaining Improved Performance Discussion with Jill.

    c. Inform Jill that there will be no need for disciplinary action.

    d. Nothing—Jill will ask for favors again if Mary remarks on her improved performance.

CHAPTER 13

DISCIPLINE AND GRIEVANCES IN THE HEALTH CARE FACILITY

INTRODUCTION

This chapter is divided into two parts.

Part One: Disciplining Nurses and Ancillary Staff

Part Two: Grievances in the Health Care Facility

Part One of this chapter is a discussion of the definition of discipline and how discipline can be approached in a positive or negative manner. We will look at how creating an atmosphere of positive discipline depends upon consistently communicating expectations with your nursing and ancillary staff. Then, we will examine the role of a nurse with supervisory duties in a facility's disciplinary procedures, emphasizing the importance of documentation. Finally, we will discuss the role that staff personal problems sometimes play in what appear to be discipline problems, and what resources nurses call on to help.

Part Two covers grievance procedures frequently used in health care facilities, and your role in grievance procedures. It will also provide you with guidelines as to how to maintain a professional attitude when someone you supervise files a grievance.

CHAPTER OBJECTIVE

After studying this chapter, you will be able to recognize the steps to disciplining staff and procedures that should be used for dealing with grievances.

LEARNING OBJECTIVES

Upon completion of this chapter, you will be able to:

1. Identify the most likely successful method for addressing disciplinary problems.

2. Specify the three questions that need to be answered when informing staff of "the rules of the game."

3. Identify the two general categories of grievances.

4. Recognize the five steps of a grievance procedure.

PART ONE—
DISCIPLINING NURSES AND ANCILLARY STAFF

In everyday usage, the word discipline has many meanings. In the organizational sense, discipline can be both positive and negative. Its definitions can include:

- Training that develops self-control, character, or orderliness and efficiency.

- Self-control or orderly conduct.

- Acceptance of direction or instruction.

- A system of rules, as for a school or a military organization.

- Treatment that corrects.

All organizations have some amount of discipline, or their work would never get done. Discipline, in the positive sense of self-control and orderly conduct, exists when all members of a group do their best to work within the rules of the organization. They see following the rules as a way to accomplish both personal and organizational objectives. Staff members as a whole should be a harmonious unit. You, as nurse supervisor, can promote positive discipline by applying the principles of effective leadership you learned in earlier units.

Discipline in the negative sense exists when people's behavior does not conform to the expected standards of acceptable conduct and some type of corrective action is required. Even then, discipline can be thought of in positive terms—a way to "make lemonade out of lemons," or to move from a less desirable condition to a more desirable one.

ACTIVITY

As a child, discipline is something your parents do to you. When you grow up, you begin to do it for yourself—discipline becomes self-discipline. On a separate piece of paper, complete the exercises described below.

1. Write briefly about a negative situation that turned out positive because you exercised self-discipline; made lemonade out of lemons. For example

   - a work situation where you received a negative appraisal and used it to improve your performance.

   - bad news from your physician that prompted you to exercise and diet.

   - a low grade in high school that prompted you to spend more time studying.

2. List a few situations in your life that require you to exercise self-discipline. For example

   - a child in your life with a diagnosed behavioral or emotional problem whose behavior is difficult to understand and accept.

   - a plateau in your performance in a favorite sport that tempts you to quit in frustration.

   - a decision to stop smoking.

   - a decision to stop giving unasked for advice.

You can probably see from your work in this activity that discipline plays an important role in the ability we have to improve our lives and our work.

COMMUNICATE YOUR EXPECTATIONS

One way to reduce the possibility of misunderstandings among staff is to clearly communicate what is expected of them. Counseling or informing your staff of "the rules of the game" can also be included in the broad scope of discipline. It is your responsibility to make sure your staff members know

WHAT is required of them by you and by the health care facility.

HOW the requirements are to be met.

WHY the requirements exist.

Imagine you have a staff member who recently started arriving 10 minutes late in the morning. In following the guidelines above for communicating your expectations, you would say

WHAT I am concerned because I have observed you arriving 10 minutes late every day for this last week. Your work day begins at 7:00 a.m.

HOW At 7:00 you should be in report, learning about the condition of the patients on the unit.

WHY It is a waste of another nurse's time to have to "fill you in" on the condition of the patients because you were late.

Communicating your expectations simply and clearly can reduce the possibility of misunderstandings.

THE CHALLENGE OF DISCIPLINE

In an ideal world, staff would follow the rules, and discipline in the negative sense would not be necessary. However, we all realize that this ideal is unrealistic. As a nurse supervisor, you will be expected to effectively deal with problem situations.

Most nurse supervisors find their experiences with discipline a challenge.

ACTIVITY

On a separate sheet of paper, list the ways that you think discipline can be challenging or difficult for nurse supervisors. Compare your list with the one below.

Some nurse supervisors have said discipline is challenging because it

- is time-consuming.

- is emotionally draining to deal with a difficult or unhappy staff member.

- requires constant changes in work priorities to concentrate on immediate problems.

- creates a feeling that the problem situation will never be resolved.

- creates a lack of trust.

- makes them feel personally responsible for problems that they cannot solve on their own.

As a supervisor, you need to remember it was the staff member who committed the unacceptable conduct, and they are responsible for their own actions. Try not to internalize the problem.

Also, remember that you are not alone. Valuable advice and guidance is available from your supervisor and the nursing department. Formal training programs in progressive discipline are recommended for new nurse supervisors.

Discipline often is a long process. Don't give up. Don't give in to the temptation to ignore the problem. Disciplinary problems you don't deal with eventually become someone else's problems.

Types of Disciplinary Actions

Discipline can be verbal or written. Discipline can be informative ("This is our policy") or punitive ("You are being demoted for your conduct").

Verbal discipline can be either informative or punitive; counseling is usually considered informative, while a verbal warning is more punitive.

DEFINITIONS

Starting with the least severe measure and working up to the most severe, disciplinary actions may take the following forms:

Counseling. Usually the first action taken; oral; clarifies standards; is documented.

Oral warning. Verbally notifies staff member that behavior or performance must be improved.

Written warning. Goes to personnel director.

Note: You may certainly discuss performance problems with a staff member without going through this formal procedure. You may have given written notice of problems that are part of an informal effort to help the staff member improve.

Reprimand. Written notification that a staff member's behavior or performance is unacceptable and that continuation or repetition of the performance may result in suspension, demotion, or removal.

Suspension. A temporary involuntary absence from work without pay for a specified period.

Transfer. Removal to a different department or work unit (used if the problem has its roots in the environment or if the staff member is clearly in the wrong job).

Demotion. Reduction to a lower level classification with a lower maximum pay or a reduction to a lower pay step in the same classification. This action remains in place indefinitely.

Removal. Permanent separation from employment.

IMPORTANT

Never indicate to a staff member that formal disciplinary measures will be invoked without first consulting with your supervisor.

THE IMPORTANCE OF DOCUMENTATION

Too often, formal disciplinary action is overturned on appeal because of the failure of nurse supervisors to document counseling efforts adequately. Refer to chapter 12 to review suggestions for counseling staff on problem behavior. Be sure to document your counseling sessions. The preferred method of documentation is the written conference memorandum. See the following "Conference Memorandum" for an example format for conference memos. Performance Reports can also be used to document counseling efforts.

CONFERENCE MEMORANDUM (PERFORMANCE STANDARD)

TO: *Staff Member's name*

FROM: *Your name*

SUBJECT: Conference of __(date)__ regarding your failure to meet performance standards/poor work habit/failure to conform to work rules.

This is to summarize our conference on the above date in_____(location)_____. That discussion and this memorandum are aimed at identifying the causes of the problem and assisting you in taking remedial action. During that conference:

A. The following items were discussed:

1. *(Cite the performance standard(s) and explain in detail how the staff member failed to meet the standard(s). Be as brief as possible, but not at the expense of specificity and clarity.)*

2.

B. You stated the following:

1.

2.

C. I offered you the following assistance and guidance:

1.

2.

D. I agreed to take the following actions by the dates indicated:

1. *(Cite actions and dates agreed to.)*

2.

E. You agreed to take the following actions by the dates indicated:

1. *(Cite actions and dates agreed to.)*

2.

Our follow-up meeting on this discussion is at _____ p.m./a.m. on _____ in _____.

If this is not an accurate summary of our conference, please notify me in writing by _____. *(Be sure to give the staff member at least three or four working days for response.)* If I do not hear from you I will assume the above to be an accurate summary.

(Optional paragraph:)

A copy of this memo will be placed in your personnel folder, which I keep in my desk. If you show improvement in this area and the problem does not recur, it will not reflect negatively in your performance report. You may add your comments to the file if you wish.

I am confident that you can improve your performance to meet or exceed the standard.

Example

Beverly has been an excellent staff nurse for five years, demonstrating good interpersonal skills. Lately, however, her head nurse, Sue, has noticed her speaking in a loud, annoying voice to her co-workers and frowning at clients when answering their questions.

Sue met with Beverly and reviewed her current performance, causes, and solutions. Beverly did not offer much information during the discussion. She just said she would not let these things happen again.

Sue was confident the problem was resolved, until the next week when she heard two nurses yelling at each other. She realized one of the nurses was Beverly. She questioned the nurses about the incident. It was a dispute over whose turn it was to answer a call light.

She met with Beverly and told her that she had noticed her smiling at clients and having friendly interactions with her co-workers. Then she asked for her reasons for this latest incident. Beverly's response was that she was "doing fine" and to "stop criticizing" her. Sue told Beverly that this kind of behavior must stop (an oral warning).

Sue's next step was to check with her manager about appropriate consequences if Beverly's behavior did not improve. She wanted to give Beverly a written warning that if she yelled at co-workers again, she would be suspended for three days. Her manager pointed out that the next step in the progressive discipline process would be a written warning that if the behavior didn't stop, severe disciplinary action would be taken.

STAFF ASSISTANCE PROGRAMS

Sometimes it becomes apparent that a disciplinary problem has its roots in a staff member's personal life. These problems may be as diverse as alcohol or drug abuse, family, marital, or behavioral disorders; they all can result in deteriorating work habits/performance.

Many health care facilities have staff assistance programs that assist staff and their dependents with personal problems.

Addictions, as well as other problems, can interfere with a staff member's ability to work. Researchers have found that

- forty percent of the American adult population marriages will end in divorce.

- three to five percent of American adults suffer from chronic, psychologically crippling forms of mental illnesses.

- fifteen percent of American adults exhibit some potentially serious symptoms of stress.

The simple fact is that problems affect nurses as well as other people, and problems affect work performance. This translates into

- absenteeism one to six times an acceptable norm.

- safety problems—15% of on-the-job accidents occur due solely to personal factors.

- escalating health and benefits costs—troubled staff members are excessive users of health and benefits plans, but are seldom treated for the real problem.

Like most nurse supervisors, you probably are not trained to diagnose alcoholism, drug addiction, or other problems. However, you are responsible for monitoring job performance and taking corrective action when necessary. Action to correct poor performance caused by personal problems is not much different from other corrective actions. **If the staff member's job performance problems are not corrected by standard disciplinary action procedures, you may need to recommend that the staff member contact an assistance program provided by the health care facility.**

Whether or not the staff member decides to accept the referral, the nurse supervisor should continue to monitor the staff member's job performance. Nurse supervisor intervention is critical if performance does not improve. You have an obligation to intervene when behavior, whatever the cause, interferes with job performance. And remember: the staff member's condition may worsen if it is ignored.

PART TWO— GRIEVANCES IN THE HEALTH CARE FACILITY

Even in the best-run health care facility units, eventually someone will become dissatisfied with his or her working conditions. It is important to give staff a quick and just means for airing and resolving their grievances. This is why many health care facilities have developed procedures to identify and resolve staff member grievances and complaints (Kozier, 1998).

Just as with performance appraisals and disciplinary actions, grievances can be handled in a positive manner. Viewed in this way, a grievance can represent an opportunity to

- use problem-solving techniques.

- create an atmosphere of trust between you and your staff.

- learn something about your style as a nurse supervisor and how it affects others.

- improve working conditions in your unit.

When a staff member files a grievance, **DO NOT** assume that

- the staff member who has filed it is a disloyal or undesirable staff member.

- there is something wrong with you, the nurse supervisor.

- everyone in your unit is unhappy.

IMPORTANT
Be careful not to make matters worse! Staff using grievance procedures should not be subject to discrimination, coercion, constraint, reprimand, or reprisal.

PURPOSE OF GRIEVANCES

There are two general categories of grievances: unfair labor practices and violations of contract. Staff who believe the health care facility has failed to provide a condition of employment guaranteed by their employment contract, or has in some way practiced unfair labor practices, may use the grievance procedure to have their allegations heard. The purpose of the grievance procedure is to encourage solving problems at the lowest possible level.

Staff filing grievances should be treated with courtesy and respect. Their allegations should be viewed seriously. Try not to feel defensive about a filed grievance. Brush up on the communications skills you learned earlier in this course.

Examples of legitimate grievances include the following:

- Consistently performing a job that requires a higher pay scale and not being compensated with the higher rate (Kozier, 1998).

- Being required to work overtime, but being told to "clock out."

- Unfair rotation of undesirable shifts (Kozier, 1998).

- Having to hold a client during x-rays.

- Lower pay scale due to gender.

- Hostile environment sexual harassment.

- Failure of the health care facility to provide gloves, gowns, or masks to care for patients in isolation.

Steps of the Grievance Procedure
STEP 1. Informal discussion with nurse supervisor

STEP 2. Formal written grievance to nurse supervisor

STEP 3. Formal meeting with staff member, management representative, and union representative

STEP 4. Arbitration

Grievance Procedure Overview

In general, grieving staff members must follow four steps, proceeding to the next step only after exhausting all resources in the current step.

The Supervisor's Role

The ability of staff and nurses in supervisory positions to talk out their problems is a time-honored method of reaching solutions together. Try not to view the grievance as a challenge to your authority. A grievance is just a problem that needs to be solved. Set aside all feelings that you are being criticized, brush up on your human relations and problem-solving skills, and get to the facts. Then

- receive the grievance objectively and unemotionally—as if the staff member were talking about someone you don't know.

- give the staff member a chance to state the whole case.

- listen—don't interrupt.

- when the staff member has finished, ask questions, but TAKE NO POSITION AT THIS TIME.

- distinguish FACTS from impressions, opinions, and hearsay.

- ask the staff member to repeat the story.

- repeat it in your own words.

- ask open-ended questions.

Sometimes, despite your best problem-solving efforts, a staff member's complaint is not settled in the first three steps and arbitration is required.

ARBITRATION

If a grievance is not resolved at Step 3, the staff member may request arbitration. When arbitration is requested, the grievance is forwarded to the labor relations office with a request to meet and attempt to resolve the dispute before submitting it to arbitration. Each labor organization has its own screening process to determine whether a grievance should be taken to arbitration. The labor relations representative will meet with the grievant and his or her representative to try to adjust the grievance. You may be contacted for background information and an explanation of your original written response.

If these efforts do not settle the grievance, the parties mutually select an arbitrator and submit a statement of the issue to the arbitrator. The arbitrator is a professional neutral whose fees are split by the health care facility and the grievant or the grievant's union.

During the hearing, you may be called upon to present testimony regarding your written response.

ACTIVITY

Sarah was hired as a staff nurse with four years experience in SICU. After passing probation, Sarah filed a grievance because her supervisor scheduled her to work four weekends in a row. In orientation she was told every nurse must work every other weekend and no more.

Sarah's supervisor, the first person Sarah notified in writing of the grievance, wrote a rebuttal explaining that nurses who had been in the health care facility for over five years were given extra weekends off, and the newer staff members were expected to work the weekends that were not covered. Sarah sent the grievance to the clinical coordinator of SICU & CCU.

1. Is this a grievable item? How do you know?

2. Is the supervisor within her rights to assign extra weekends to newer staff?

Activity Feedback

1. Yes, this is a condition of work and is a grievable item.

2. No, the supervisor has no right to assign extra weekends to new staff unless they volunteer.

EXAM QUESTIONS

CHAPTER 13
Questions 96–100

96. What three questions need to be answered when a supervisor is informing a staff member of the "rules of the game?"

    a. how long, when, why

    b. what, how, why

    c. how much, what, how long

    d. who, when, why

97. What method of addressing disciplinary problems usually taken first?

    a. written warnings

    b. oral warnings

    c. performance reports

    d. counseling

Question 98 refers to the situation described in the paragraph below.

Linda is a nurse in the Cardiac Care Unit. Linda's supervisor Cindy has assigned her the most difficult patient on the Unit for two weeks straight. Cindy always compliments Linda on being one of her most competent staff members. Linda does not want to continue to take the most difficult patients, and feels she is being discriminated against because of her strong work ethic.

98. What is the next step Linda should take?

    a. Write a formal written grievance to the supervising nurse.

    b. Arrange an informal discussion with the supervising nurse.

    c. Arrange a formal meeting with the unit supervisor and a union representative.

    d. Write a request for arbitration.

99. Ann believes her nurse supervisor has failed to live up to the requirements of her employee contract. She has met with the supervisor and feels dissatisfied with the results. What is her next step?

    a. arbitration

    b. formal written grievance to her nurse supervisor

    c. formal written grievance to department head

    d. informal discussion with her nurse supervisor

100. What are the two general categories of grievances?

    a. wage disputes and unfair hiring practices

    b. discriminatory practices and Nurse Practice Act violations

    c. unfair labor practices and violations of contracts

    d. poor management and unsafe work conditions

GLOSSARY

Arbitration - The hearing and determining of a dispute or the settling of differences between parties by a person or persons chosen or agreed to by them.

Authoritarian management - A style of management favoring complete obedience or subjection to authority as opposed to individual freedom: authoritarian principles; authoritarian attitudes.

Categorize - To arrange in categories or classes; classify. To describe by labeling or giving a name to; characterize.

Client - The recipient of nursing care, including the prevention of illness or the promotion of care.

Character defense - A personality trait, as a habitual tendency to idealize or rationalize, that serves some unconscious defensive purpose.

Conflict - To come into collision or disagreement; be contradictory, at variance, or in opposition.

Cooperation - An act or instance of working or acting together for a common purpose or benefit. More or less active assistance from a person, or group. Activity shared for mutual benefit.

Compromise - A settlement of differences by mutual concessions; an agreement reached by adjustment of conflicting or opposing claims, principles, etc., by reciprocal modification of demands.

Committee - A person or group of persons elected or appointed to perform some service or function, as to investigate, report on, or act upon a particular matter.

Communication - The act or process of communicating; fact of being communicated. The imparting or interchange of thoughts, opinions, or information by speech, writing, or other media.

Communication environment - The physical surroundings in which communication takes place. Environments can range from a quiet office to a noisy emergency room to a playing field in a park.

Culture - A view of the world and set of traditions by a particular group that are transmitted from generation to generation.

Direction - The act or an instance of directing. Providing management, control, guidance, and supervision.

Delegate - To send or appoint (a person) as deputy or representative to perform a duty or task. To commit (powers, functions, etc.) to another.

Denial - An unconscious defense mechanism used to reduce anxiety by denying thoughts, feelings, or facts that are consciously intolerable.

Disorganization - The absence of organization or orderly arrangement; disarrangement; disorder.

Equal Opportunity - Policies and practices in employment and other areas that do not discriminate against persons on the basis of race, color, religion, sex, age, mental or physical handicap, or national origin.

Feedback - A response to a message. When you give feedback, you relay your feelings about or understanding of a message you received. When you ask for feedback, you are checking to see whether your message was received as you intended.

Formal norms - The way people conduct themselves in carrying out their jobs or interacting with others due to accepted workplace policies or standards written for that institution or industry.

Goal - The result or achievement toward which effort is directed; aim; end.

Grievance - A wrong considered as grounds for complaint, or something believed to cause distress. A complaint or resentment, as against an unjust or unfair act.

Halo effect - A predisposition to admire all of a person's actions, work, etc., because of an estimable quality or action in the past. A potential inaccuracy in observation, as of a person, due to overgeneralization from a limited amount of evidence or the influence of preconceived beliefs.

Incident report - A record of an accident or incident created for the health care facility.

Informal norms - The way people conduct themselves in carrying out their jobs or interacting with others due to accepted behaviors adopted by persons in that institution or industry. These adopted behaviors are not backed up by written policies.

Informal organizations - Consists of the relationships among the formal organization's members. The power of the informal organization lies in its unwritten rules, or organizational norms. These unwritten rules come about through the pressures brought to bear by the relationships of co-workers.

Interview - A face to face meeting in which two or more persons meet to discuss a job opening. The goal of the discussion is for the person applying for the job to learn more about the workplace and the job duties, and for the interviewer to evaluate the applicant for satisfactory qualifications.

Manager - The person who carries out policies, regulations and rules of an organization, with the official authority to act.

Meditation - The act of meditating. Continued or extended thought; reflection; contemplation.

Message - A piece of information. The message you intend to send may or may not be the message that is received; use feedback to check.

Motivation - The intention of achieving a goal, leading to goal-directed behavior. A motive is defined as an innate force modified by learning that serves to satisfy needs that are not directly tied to the body requirements.

Objective - An objective is the description of a performance you want the students to be able to exhibit before you consider them competent.

On-the-job training - Job skills received, or happening while in actual performance of one's work.

One-way communication - Communication that goes from the sender to the receiver only - there is no opportunity for a response or a question form the receiver.

Orientation - The formal process of teaching a new employee about the health care facility and that employee's job function in the facility.

Organization - A functional group such as a health care facility that allocates the people and resources who work toward achieving goals.

Organizational norms - These are standard, currently accepted methods of doing things in an organization. They are specific guides to conduct and provide a way for individuals to organize and structure their behavior.

Perception - The act or faculty of discovering by means of the senses or of the mind, cognition, and understanding. The immediate or intuitive recognition or appreciation, as of moral, psychological, or aesthetic qualities. A single unified awareness derived from sensory processes while a stimulus is present.

Perceptual filters - The ways in which each of us distorts messages. The negative consequence of our perceptual filters is balanced by feedback, which corrects the misunderstandings caused by our filters.

Performance appraisals - A formal way for a supervisor to give feedback to a staff member concerning their performance on the job. They help the staff member clarify new responsibilities that have evolved in their job, and help supervisors provide frank and constructive feedback to the staff member.

Performance discrepancy - The difference between what is being done on the job and what is supposed to be done.

Physical barriers to communication - Physical barriers are environmental factors that block communication. Physical barriers include noise level, distance between sender and receiver, and too much or too little light.

Prejudice - An unfavorable opinion or feeling formed beforehand or without knowledge, thought, or reason. Any preconceived opinion or feeling, either favorable or unfavorable; especially those opinions of a hostile nature, regarding a racial, religious, or national group.

Problem solving - The problem solving process includes the identification of the problem and then seeking alternative actions that will solve the problem.

Progressive discipline - A series of steps taken when an employee's behavior becomes chronically disruptive. The behavior is documented and the employee must witness the documentation. A plan is created with the employee to change the behavior. Follow-up meetings are held and behavior changes are monitored.

Projection - The tendency to ascribe to another person feelings, thoughts, or attitudes present in oneself, or to regard external reality as embodying such feelings, thoughts, etc., in some way.

Rationalize - To ascribe (one's acts, opinions, etc.) to causes that superficially seem reasonable and valid but that actually are unrelated to the true, possibly unconscious and often less creditable or agreeable causes.

Receiver - A person who hears a message communicated by a sender.

Reflection - The act of reflecting or the state of being reflected. A fixing of the thoughts on something; careful consideration.

Resources - The people, money, equipment, facilities, and supplies available to do a job or complete a project.

Role - A set of behaviors that is organized and attributed to functioning in a specific job or position.

Screening - The act or work of a person who screens, as in ascertaining the character and competence of applicants, employees, etc.

Self-image - The idea, conception, or mental image one has of oneself.

Sender - A person who relays a message to a receiver. The sender and receiver roles reverse many times during a given exchange.

Staff - A group of persons, as employees, charged with carrying out the work of an establishment or executing some undertaking.

Staffing - A system of assigning personnel to fill the nursing roles needed to carry out client care in a health care facility.

Stereotype - A simplified and standardized conception or image invested with special meaning and held in common by members of a group. To characterize or regard as a stereotype.

Stress - A specific response by the body to a stimulus, as fear or pain, that disturbs or interferes with the normal physiological equilibrium of an organism. Any physical, mental, or emotional strain or tension, or a situation, occurrence, or factor causing these states.

Supervisor - A person who directs and oversees workers, or the work done by others.

Task force - A group or committee, usually of experts or specialists, formed for analyzing, investigating, or solving a specific problem.

Team - People joined in a group for a cooperative effort or special purpose.

Two-way communication - Communication in which there is opportunity for the sender and the receiver to interact. The receiver may respond and question the sender about what is being said.

Values - Values is the relative worth, merit, or importance of something. The ideals, customs, institutions, etc., of a society toward which the people of the group have an affective regard. To consider with respect to worth, excellence, usefulness, or importance.

Withdrawal - To remove oneself from some activity, competition, etc.

Witness - A person who sees, hears, or knows by personal presence and perception: to witness an event. To attest by one's signature.

BIBLIOGRAPHY

Bradley, J. C. & Edinberg, M. A. (1990). *Communication in the Nursing Context* (3rd ed.). Norwalk, CT: Appleton & Lange.

Chapman, E. N. (1995). *Attitude: Your Most Priceless Possession.* Los Altos, CA: Crisp Publications, Inc.

Charlesworth, E. A. & Nathan, R. G. (1991). *Stress Management: A Comprehensive Guide to Wellness.* New York: Ballantine Books.

Daniels, W. R. (1990). Group Power II: A Manager's Guide to Conducting Regular Meetings. San Diego: University Associates, Inc.

Deloughery, G. (Ed.). (1998). *Issues and Trends in Nursing* (3rd ed.). Baltimore: Mosby Year Book Inc.

Douglas, L. M. (1996). *The Effective Nurse Manager* (5th ed.). St. Louis: Mosby Year Book.

Finch, L. (1995). *Telephone Courtesy & Customer Service* (2nd ed.). Los Altos, CA: Crisp Publications.

Fisher, M. L. (1996). *Quick Reference to Redesigning the Nursing Organization.* Albany, NY: Delmar Publishers.

Flarey, D. L. (1995). *Redesigning Nursing Care Delivery: Transforming Our Future* (2nd ed.). Philadelphia: J. B. Lippincott Co.

Fuller, G. (1995). *Supervisor's Portable Answer Book* (2nd ed.). New Jersey: Prentice Hall, Inc.

Kozier, B. (1998). *Fundamentals of Nursing: Concepts, Process, and Practice* (5th ed.). Menlo Park, CA: Addison Wesley Longman, Inc.

Maddux, R. (1997). *Team Building: An Exercise in Leadership* (Rev. ed). Los Altos, CA: Crisp Publications.

Mager, R. & Pipe, P. (1997). *Analyzing Performance Problems, or, You really oughta wanna: how to figure out why people aren't doing what they should be, and what to do about it* (3rd ed. Rev.). Atlanta: Center for Effective Performance.

Mager, R. F. (1997). *Measuring Instructional Results or Got a Match?* (3rd ed., Rev.). Atlanta: Center for Effective Performance.

Mager, R. (1997). *Goal Analysis: how to clarify your goals so you can actually achieve them* (3rd ed., Rev.). Atlanta: Center for Effective Performance.

Marrelli, T. M. (1997). *The Nurse Manager's Survival Guide: Practical Answers to Everyday Problems* (2nd ed.). St. Louis: Mosby Year Book, Inc.

Mills, J. (1992). *Coping with Stress: A Guide to Living.* New York: John Wiley & Sons, Inc.

Porter-O'Grady, T. (Ed.). (1994). *The Nurse Manager's Problem Solver.* St. Louis: Mosby Year Book, Inc.

Potter, B. (1995). *Preventing Job Burnout.* Los Altos, CA: Crisp Publications, Inc.

Pugh, M. (1997). *Nurse Manager—A Practical Guide to Better Employee Relations.* Philadelphia: W. B. Saunders Co.

Swansburg, R. C. (1996). *Management and Leadership for Nurse Managers* (2nd ed.). Boston: Jones and Bartlett Publishers.

Sullivan, M. (1994). *Nursing Leadership and Management.* Springhouse, PA: Springhouse Corporation.

Tappen, R. M. (1995). *Nursing leadership and management: concepts and practice* (3rd ed.). Philadelphia: F.A. Davis.

INDEX

PRETEST KEY

Supervisory Skills for Nurses

1.	B	Chapter 1
2.	C	Chapter 2
3.	B	Chapter 2
4.	D	Chapter 8
5.	D	Chapter 2
6.	A	Chapter 10
7.	C	Chapter 11
8.	C	Chapter 12
9.	B	Chapter 3
10.	C	Chapter 3
11.	A	Chapter 3
12.	B	Chapter 4
13.	A	Chapter 5
14.	B	Chapter 4
15.	A	Chapter 9
16.	D	Chapter 13
17.	A	Chapter 7
18.	B	Chapter 6

Western Schools® offers over 60 topics to suit all your interests – and requirements!

Clinical Conditions/Nursing Practice

A Nurse's Guide to Weight Control
for Healthy Living......................................25 hrs
Auscultation Skills: Breath and Heart Sounds ......12 hrs
Basic Nursing of Head, Chest, Abdominal,
Spine and Orthopedic Trauma ....16 hrs
Cancer Nursing: A Solid Foundation for Practice ..30 hrs
Care at the End of Life.......................................3 hrs
Chemotherapy Essentials: Principles & Practice ..15 hrs
Chest Tube Management ....2 hrs
Diabetes Nursing Care.......................................30 hrs
Healing Nutrition ....24 hrs
Hepatitis C: The Silent Killer ....2 hrs
HIV/AIDS.......................................1, 2, 4 or 30 hrs
Holistic & Complementary Therapies: Introduction..1 hr
Influenza: A Vaccine-Preventable Disease ....1 hr
Managing Obesity and Eating Disorders ....30 hrs
Pain Management: Principles and Practice............30 hrs
Popular Diets and Diet Drugs ....2 hrs
Practical Weight Control: Assessment & Planning..7 hrs
Practical Weight Control: Lifestyle Interventions..10 hrs
Pressure Ulcers: Guidelines for Prevention
and Nursing Management................................30 hrs
The Neurological Exam.......................................1 hr

Critical Care/ER/OR

Ambulatory Surgical Care ....20 hrs
Case Studies in Critical Care Nursing:
A Guide for Application and Review ....36 hrs
Principles of Basic Trauma Nursing ....30 hrs

Geriatrics

Alzheimer's: Things a Nurse Needs to Know........12 hrs
Elder Abuse ....4 hrs
Home Health Nursing ....30 hrs
Major Issues in Gerontological Nursing ....10 hrs
Nursing Care of the Older Adult ....30 hrs

Hot Topics/Issues

Belt Lipectomy: Lower Body Contouring ....1 hr
Biological Weapons ....5 hrs
Botox Treatments and Dermal Fillers.......................1 hr
Influenza: A Vaccine-Preventable Disease ....1 hr
SARS: An Emerging Public Health Threat ....1 hr
Smallpox..2 hrs
The New Threat of Drug Resistant Microbes ....5 hrs
Weight Loss Surgery ....1 hr
West Nile Virus ....1 hr

Maternal-Child/Pediatrics/Women's Health

Attention Deficit Hyperactivity Disorders
Throughout the Lifespan.................................30 hrs
Caring for Women: Selected Topics ....7 hrs
Challenges in Women's Health: PMS;
Reproductive Choices; Menopause;
Gynecological Disorders ....2-5 hrs
Child Abuse ....30 hrs
End-of-Life Care for Children and
Their Families ....2 hrs
IPV (Intimate Partner Violence):
A Domestic Violence Concern ....1 or 3 hrs
Manual of School Health....................................30 hrs
Maternal-Newborn Nursing.................................30 hrs
Pediatric Nursing: Routine to Emergent Care........30 hrs
Pediatric Pharmacology ....10 hrs
Pediatric Physical Assessment.............................10 hrs
Women's Health: Contemporary
Advances and Trends ....30 hrs

Professional Issues/Management/Law

Medical Error Prevention: Patient Safety ....2 hrs
Nursing Ethics and the Law..................................30 hrs
Nursing and Malpractice Risks:
Understanding the Law ....30 hrs
Ohio Law: Standards of Safe Nursing Practice ....1 hr
Supervisory Skills for Nurses ....30 hrs
Surviving and Thriving in Nursing ....30 hrs
Understanding Managed Care...............................30 hrs

Psychiatric/Mental Health

Basic Psychopharmacology....................................5 hrs
Child Abuse ....30 hrs
IPV (Intimate Partner Violence):
A Domestic Violence Concern ....1 or 3 hrs
Psychiatric Principles & Applications for
General Patient Care ....30 hrs
Psychiatric Nursing Update: Current Trends
in Diagnosing and Treatment ....30 hrs
Substance Abuse ....30 hrs

Visit us online at www.westernschools.com for these great courses – plus all the latest CE topics!
Online testing also available.

REV. 1/04

Made in the USA
Middletown, DE
22 March 2023

27424714R00027